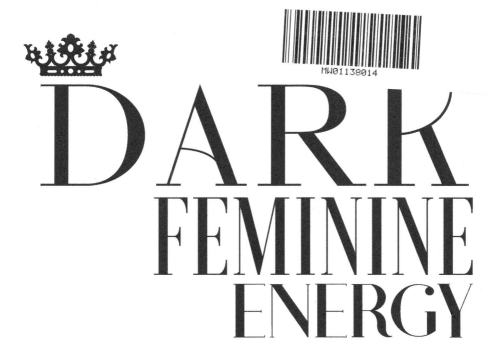

DARK
FEMININE
ENERGY

The Complete Guide to Channel Your Inner Femme Fatale.
Learn Self-Reflection, Self-Compassion, Master the Male
Psyche, and Develop a Magnetic Body Language

EMILY REACHER

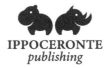

IPPOCERONTE
publishing

Book Formatting designed by macrovector, rawpixel.com from Freepik, and thiwwy design,
Cover designed by thiwwy design (@thiwwy)

CONTENTS

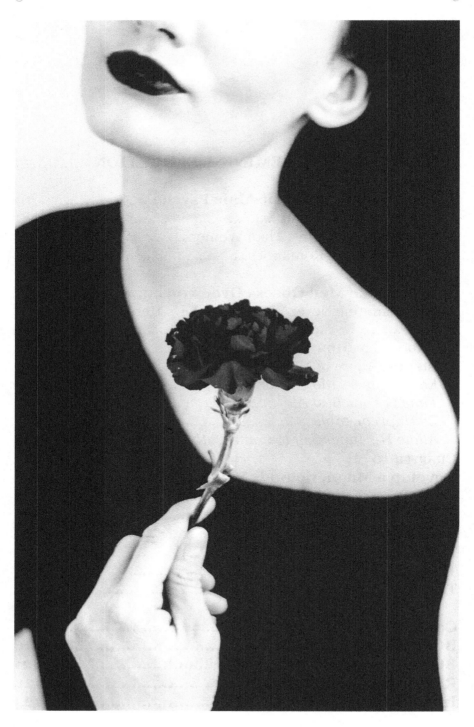

Introduction

In the modern world, having healthy relationships, stopping people from stepping on you, and being able to relate to others positively and constructively is not easy. For many women, it is challenging to be assertive, put their interests and desires ahead of others, and build relationships of mutual respect.

It's not their fault; it depends on how our society works. Unfortunately, being too good doesn't pay; the world is full of people ready to take advantage of a moment of weakness.

Think for a moment of call centers or door-to-door salespeople, ready to make us buy their products by any means, or guys in a bar who would say anything to get a girl to bed that night. As women, we naturally must learn to protect ourselves, not with physical strength, but with our minds.

I wrote this book for women who want to take control of their lives, those who have loved and suffered, those who want to be respected both at work and in private, and those who wish to have the weapons to win in life.

I wrote the book I wish I had read when I was younger, before starting my coaching career. In my youth, I always had trouble getting the respect I deserved; I was shy and too good, and more than once, I gave in to pressure from my peers.

With these pages, I will teach you how to avoid making my mistakes and how to tune in to your dark feminine energy.

As a result, you will learn to become more assertive, seduce with your magnetic personality, gain the respect you deserve, and become a true femme fatale.

When I talk about femme fatale, I'm not referring to the extreme version that we see in the movies, the one that leads men to their ruin. Instead, I'm talking about a woman who knows what she wants, how to get it, and how to take leadership in a relationship by putting her needs first.

The path that I have structured with this book could be atypical, but I am also convinced that it is the one that gives the best results.

This volume is divided into three parts:

- The *first part* provides any reader with the **theoretical basis** for understanding what dark and light feminine energies are and how they relate to the figure of the femme fatale.

- The *second part* focuses on **yourself and how to access your dark feminine energy**. It offers a series of approaches to finding your balance and gaining confidence. It creates the foundation for feeling comfortable in the role of the femme fatale.

- The *third part* will teach you to **behave like a femme fatale** and to **relate to men and the world around you**.

I realize that many of you would be tempted to skip ahead to part three, but in my personal experience, it is tough to access your dark feminine energy without first working on yourself. When you have found your balance and confidence, that's the time to start looking outside of yourself.

Without further ado, let's start our journey by talking about what dark feminine energy is and how it can help us in our everyday lives!

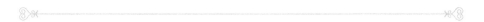

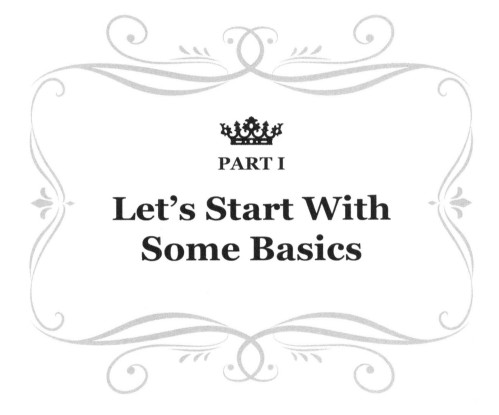

PART I

Let's Start With Some Basics

CHAPTER 1

What is the Dark Feminine Energy?

Think like a queen. A queen is not afraid to fail. Failure is another steppingstone to greatness.
—Oprah Winfrey

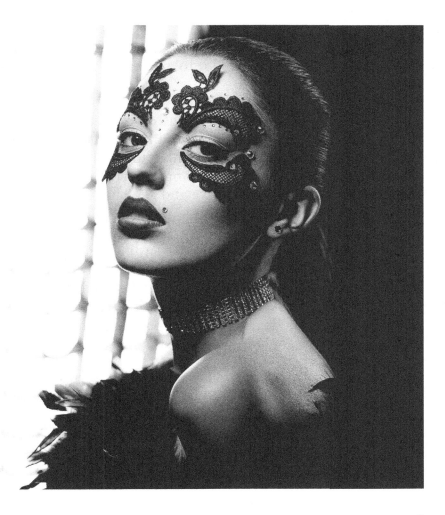

Dark feminine energy is a widely used term in the spiritual community, but it might be a foreign term or even sound dangerous for people not part of this circle. In truth, dark feminine energy can be understood as one-half of the spectrum of femininity. This energy includes aspects that are frowned upon by religion and society.

We can break the feminine spectrum into two parts: dark and light. Using an analogy, we can compare the spectrum of femininity to two beautiful horses: white and black. The white horse is the one that everyone picks, but the dark is equally beautiful, full of mystery, and much more fascinating.

Dark feminine energy is the opposite of light feminine energy; it is a part of us, and we need it to express our full potential as women.

The dark feminine is one-half of the divine feminine. It is not the negative, evil aspect of the feminine but rather the dark, fiery, transformational aspect of womanhood. The dark feminine is our rare, exquisite, and uncommon part. It's the energy we can draw on to be more assertive and get what we want without leaning on our masculine energy.

The dark feminine energy is the part we keep hidden for fear of judgment since, over the centuries, our patriarchal and religious society has pushed us to believe it could be wrong and harmful. In this book, we will explore this type of energy from different angles and learn to love who we are, embracing every side of our power, including the one that used to be rejected.

Another point worth discussing is the concept of "dark." So many aspects of our being are rarely used. This happens because we are unaware of our full potential or are not used to thinking in specific ways. What's in the shadows isn't necessarily evil, and "dark" doesn't necessarily have a negative connotation; it all depends on how you use it.

Duality is a recurring theme in the Catholic religion. Christ is the lion and the lamb, God is the judge and the father, and the Virgin Mary is both mother and virgin. Yet, even in the Holy Spirit, there is a duality; it can be gentle and powerful. Religion has taught us to accept these dualities, so why should we deny the duality in women or hide it? The dark feminine is part of us and should be accepted and explored instead of dismissed.

The dark feminine is the aspect that pertains to desire, passion, and sexuality. Again, we see examples of this aspect used in multiple fields, from Hollywood movies to advertising; anyone who uses dark feminine energy to get what they want.

Think of Angelina Jolie, Rihanna, Lady Gaga, Beyoncé, Marilyn Monroe, and many more.

All of these celebrities have some traits in common. They are all successful, empowered, self-confident women wrapped in an aura of mystery and for whom men would go crazy. Aesthetic beauty is an essential factor of attraction, but that's not all; and for many men, it even takes second place compared to other characteristics. Most men crave the dark feminine in their women as much as the light feminine, perhaps even more. When something is rare, it has more value, and given how few women embrace this side of their personality, these women have enormous value.

Accepting our darker side doesn't mean becoming Morticia Addams. There are moments and appropriate places to give space to what is in the shadows and moments in which it is good to stay in the light. For example, bringing out our dark side while flirting with a single man can be fun, but relating in the same way with someone's husband can become problematic. On the other hand, moving from passive to dominant in bed can rekindle the spark of a dormant relationship in couples who have been married for a long time. Finding the right balance is vital to success and achieving what we want.

Balance is necessary for all aspects of our spirituality and our physical reality. However, as much as we need to balance our feminine and masculine energies, we must also balance our dark and light feminine.

The dark feminine is not only about sensuality and desire; there are other reasons why we desperately need it. The light feminine is characterized by being lovable, free, laid back, and chill. Unfortunately, these characteristics often attract players, abusers, losers, and those who want to exploit our weaknesses for their interests.

These people expect you to tolerate disrespect, indifference, or being neglected.

Luckily, the dark feminine in us does not tolerate such behaviors. This is one of the reasons why accessing this side of our personality is essential; it allows us to protect ourselves and avoid these unpleasant situations.

We are drawn to the dark as well. Think for a moment about those men who are in tune with their dark masculinity. We cannot push them around or take them for granted since they might walk away if we disrespect them. However, when a man channels his dark masculinity, he can act as a gentleman but not be taken for a ride; he has an element of danger that is part of his intoxicating personality.

The dark feminine is quite similar; she can be loving and caring but at the same time will not tolerate any nonsense from any man at any time. This does not mean having an aggressive or violent attitude; the dark feminine is constantly supported by healthy self-esteem and a sense of self-worth. She is assertive, asking gently but firmly for what she wants, and enjoying the pleasures of life by putting herself ahead of others. Again, this doesn't mean being self-centered but knowing how to recognize your own value and not be belittled by others.

The dark feminine has a healthy relationship with her wants and needs; she is not driven by shame, guilt, or fear; instead, she speaks up, communicating her standards without fearing losing a man.

So, to put it plain and simple; a woman in tune with her dark feminine energy knows who she is, she understands her desires and quickly gets what she wants because of her magnetic personality.

CHAPTER 2
The Femme Fatale

Good girls go to heaven, bad girls go everywhere.
—Mae West

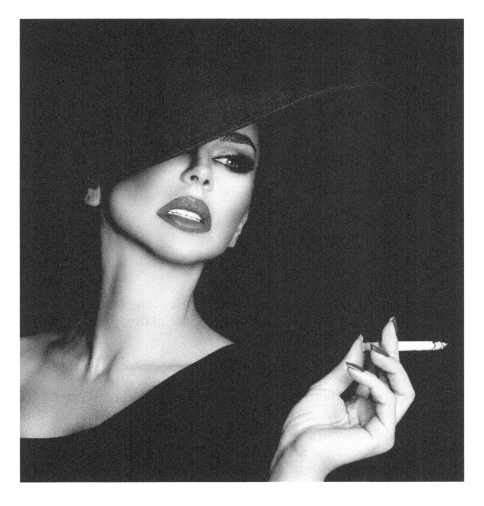

The femme fatale is an ancient female archetype found in the myths and folklore of many cultures. It became popular with classic film noir of the 1940s and '50s; she earned her name; French for "fatal woman" because she traditionally brings about the man's destruction. She is magnetic, seductive, and irresistible, and often makes a stunning first impression.

The femme fatale in movies and books uses her sexuality as a tool to get what she wants. In addition, she likes money, material things, and carnal pleasure and has a cynical view of the world. For these reasons, in most works of fiction, she is presented as an ambivalent character leaning toward the dark side.

The femme fatale is powerful *because* she is a woman, not despite it.

Modern examples of a femme fatale in popular culture are:

- Poison Ivy, from the *Batman Series*, with her seductive red lips but poisonous kiss
- Jessica Rabbit from *Who Framed Roger Rabbit*
- Madeleine Elster in *Vertigo*
- Eva Green in *Sin City: A Dame to Kill For*
- Isabella Rossellini in *Fatal Attraction*

The list is just endless. Also, you can find many celebrities who give "femme fatale vibes" daily, even if social media has recently taken away some of their aura of mystery.

The critical thing to understand is that the figure of the femme fatale was born from the mind of male authors. The figures presented in fiction are mostly unrealistic and would not work well in the real world. However, the femme fatale has had enormous success because these authors give voice to a male need to relate to a strong, independent female figure.

For many psychologists who study popular culture, the femme fatale is nothing more than the fictionalized and extreme version of the alpha or dominant woman, studied for the first time in 1939 by Maslow.

Monika K. Sumra, in her paper *Masculinity, femininity, and leadership:Taking a closer look at the alpha female*, summarized Maslow's idea:

> *High-dominant women would make great leaders, though not every dominant woman would become one. [...] They are rarely embarrassed, self-conscious, shy, or fearful compared to women who were not dominant (low-dominant feeling).[...] Dominant women have more self-confidence, higher poise, prefer to be treated like a "person" and not like a "woman," prefer independence and "standing on their own feet," lack feelings of inferiority, and generally do not care for concessions that imply they are inferior, weak, or that they need special attention and cannot take care of themselves (2019).*

We can see that most of the characteristics listed by Maslow are traits of the femme fatale archetype. The femme fatale is, therefore, an "amplified" alpha woman to the point of becoming utterly irresistible to the men who surround her. This figure embodies multiple male sexual fantasies, so it works so well in films and books, but of course, it wouldn't work the same in real life.

I know, I know, this book promises in the title to make you a femme fatale. But the goal is not to become a caricature of some fictional character or make you a completely different person. Instead, I want to teach you how to use certain valuable traits of the femme fatale in some situations. To do this, I will show you how to access your dark feminine energy when needed. It is essential to understand that using only your dark feminine energy 100% of the time inevitably leads to developing toxic femininity. So, you want to find the right mix of light and dark feminine energy instead. Simply put, you might want to be the femme fatale on a first date, but you don't want to be one when you're at grandma's for lunch.

CHAPTER 3
Light and Dark Feminine Energies

Above all, be the heroine of your life, not the victim.
—Nora Ephron

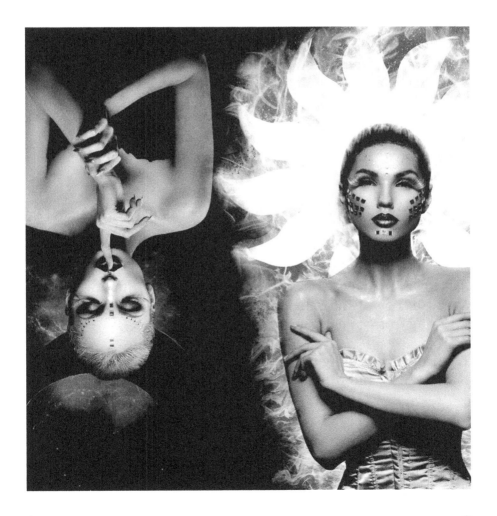

Before explaining the differences between light and dark feminine energy, I want to clarify the difference between feminine and masculine energy. I consider this explanation necessary because many people often confuse dark feminine energy with masculine energy.

Masculine energy is about logic, initiative, and pursuing goals. It is the energy that drives us to action to apply changes in the outside world so that we can fit better. Playing sports and making plans are actions that stimulate our masculine energy. When the masculine energy is too intense, it can manifest itself through control, manipulation, and, worst cases, violence.

The feminine energy dwells on internal emotions and manifestation. Instead of actions, it focuses on being and receiving. Creativity, self-care, and acceptance are aspects of feminine energy. When this energy is wounded, it leads to self-isolation and a lack of confidence.

Each individual possesses both, masculine and feminine, energies but one tends to prevail.

Now that we have clarified the differences between these two energies, we can discuss in detail the feminine one.

Light and dark feminine energies are two faces of the same medal. However, most women tend towards the light side, mainly because society and religion influence our personality in a certain way from an early age.

Light feminine energy is the embodiment of our society's traditional values and promotes qualities like being:
- nurturing
- intuitive
- affectionate
- compassionate

- forgiving
- empathetic
- peaceful
- positive
- supportive
- pure
- emotional

We can see how these qualities align with our society's traditional values and how a woman with all these traits is seen as a perfect potential wife, homemaker, caregiver, etc.

Dark feminine energy, as already mentioned, is opposed, and sometimes characterized by a negative connotation. However, the truth is that this energy is not harmful, and if used correctly, it can be our precious ally.

Some women use it purely for manipulative purposes; in that case, it becomes toxic femininity. Others, with some practice, find the right balance between the two energies and drastically improve their lives.

A woman in tune with her dark feminine energy is:

- assertive
- passionate
- mysterious
- seductive
- authentic
- powerful
- magnetic
- private
- dominant

Let's see some of them in more detail.

Mysterious: A woman that masters her dark feminine energy is often defined as mysterious. But what does it mean to be mysterious? Think about a woman who does not overshare, she keeps to herself, and you will never know who she is unless you closely connect with her. The mystery is highly seductive. It may seem like a trivial thing to say, but it is the reality, and several studies in this regard support this thesis.

Mysteries attract us because we are naturally curious beings, and when we have incomplete information, we want to fill the gap and find out as much as possible.

> *Humans are known to seek non-instrumental information, or become 'curious' about such information, such as answers to obscure trivia questions, or celebrity gossip that will have little future value. People's curiosity for non-instrumental information is also illustrated in the fact that people will pay or exert effort to access information. For example, one might pay for a subscription to a gossip magazine or wait in line to buy tickets to watch a documentary film, in the knowledge that the information provided will not hold instrumental value (FitzGibbon, 2020).*

It is, therefore, natural that a woman who keeps her best secrets to herself is a source of interest and curiosity.

Humble: You might think that for a woman in tune with her dark feminine energy, bragging is a natural part of her magnetic personality. However, it is precisely the opposite; She does not want to boast of her successes but invites people to discover her little by little. Likewise, she does not brag or overshare on social media to keep her aura of mystery intact.

Being humble adds to her personality. Also, it elevates her above all the people jostling desperately to be in the spotlight for a few seconds.

Private: Women who have learned to master their dark feminine energy are not intimate with many people. Instead, they keep a few trusted friends and family close and surround themselves with only high-value people.

They do not want to share their energy with people who are negative or not worth spending time with. They know whom they want and are not afraid to draw the line.

Passionate: Another trait is being passionate. This does not refer only to the sexual sphere but to one's own interests. Women who have learned to master their dark feminine energy have many interests and are unafraid to try new things.

Discussing their passions with them is a source of inspiration. You can hear from their words how much they care about what they do, and thanks to their magnetic personality, you want to know more and more.

Authentic: Women who know how to tap into their dark feminine energy are often called authentic. This is because they rarely sweeten the pill.

As I have already said, they are not talkative; what they say is always polite and straightforward. They speak their mind even at the cost of hurting someone's feelings.

They are true to their personality, values, and spirit, regardless of the pressure that they are under to act otherwise.

Powerful: Being powerful, more than a trait in itself, is the combination of all the previous ones. A strong, assertive woman who knows what she wants and how to get it automatically conveys a sense of power.

To understand what I'm talking about, think of some celebrities who use dark feminine energy as their secret weapon: Angelina Jolie, Mariah Carey, P!nk, and many others. All of them are extremely powerful and successful women. But have you ever wondered what would happen if someone took away all their money, fame, and material goods? Men would still fall at their feet, and they would still be popular. It is undeniable that money and success allow you to influence people, but the real power is something else. True power is within us, and not everyone knows how to access it.

As you can see, the traits associated with the dark feminine energy are very different from those of its light counterpart. So, now you are probably wondering, when should I use my dark side and why? Isn't light feminine energy enough to move forward in life?

In some cases, the light feminine energy is not enough; relationships with men are a perfect example. Men use dark masculine energy when trying to get something from us when we are not cooperating. When men tap into this energy, they may assume an aggressive stance meant to let us know they are in a dominant position at that moment. Instead of using their energy to make us feel safe, they use it to get the better of us and get what they want.

By this, I do not mean that dark masculine energy is necessarily associated with verbal or physical violence. Instead, it is simply a change of attitude in the male to try to assert his point of view. However, if a man begins to operate using only his dark masculine energy to get what he wants, then he becomes toxic masculinity. When a person enters a prolonged state of toxic masculinity, it is no longer a question of which energy to use; leaving is the best choice.

However, when we see a man using his dark masculinity energy to get what he wants from us, we can react with the right tools.

Light feminine energy will not work well in these situations. Instead, channeling our dark feminine energy will help us to be assertive and not let him get his way.

My clients usually smile at this point, thinking it is easier said than done.

Do not worry if you do not know where to start; in the following chapters, you will see how to draw on your dark feminine energy and deal with this and other situations. You will learn battle-tested tips and tricks from strong, successful women and how to change the perception that others have of you while remaining yourself.

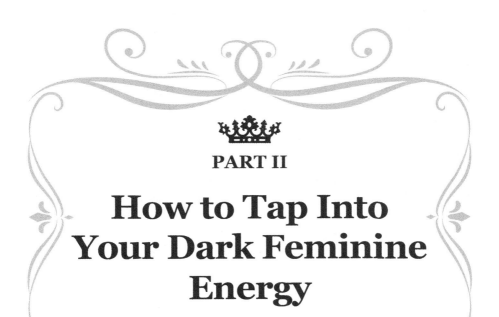

PART II

How to Tap Into Your Dark Feminine Energy

From now on, we will start to get serious; if the book's first part were just basics, I will share practical advice to access a new side of yourself from this section.

You first need to know that most exercises we will do are mental. These are the most critical part of the book. Of course, the look and the attitude have their weight, but it all starts in your mind. Some people believe it is enough to wear high heels, more aggressive clothing, and act confidently to access their dark feminine energy. Unfortunately, it rarely works. Otherwise, it would be too easy, and everyone could do it. It is like building a house without a solid foundation. It may stand for a while, and many may admire its beauty, but in the long run, it is bound to collapse.

What I want you to do instead is work on yourself. I will help you to fill the gap between who you are inside and who you appear to be outside. Remember that an essential characteristic of dark feminine is being authentic. Otherwise, taking acting lessons and pretending to be whomever you want would be enough.

Instead, I want you to become "the whole package." So, at the end of this book and with some practice, you will be able to channel your inner femme fatale when needed, but also switch modes and use your light feminine energy if the case requires it.

It is important to remember that everyone's experience of their dark feminine energy is unique and personal and that there is no one right way to tap into it. Therefore, be mindful and gentle with yourself as you explore this aspect, and always prioritize your safety and wellbeing.

CHAPTER 4

Practice Self-Care

The way I see it, if you want the rainbow, you gotta put up with the rain!
−Dolly Parton

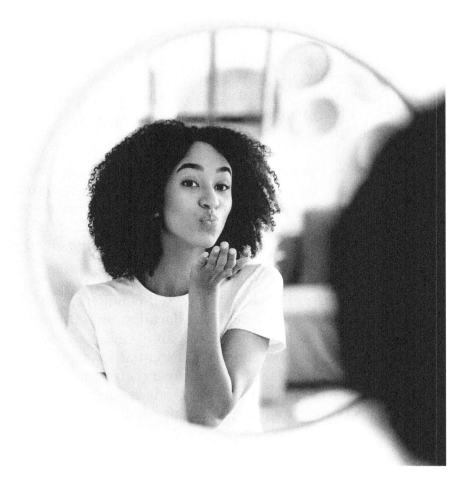

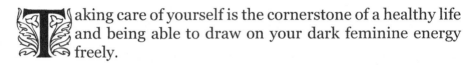

aking care of yourself is the cornerstone of a healthy life and being able to draw on your dark feminine energy freely.

Self-care is important at all stages of life and health status to promote wellbeing, prevent disease, and improve health outcomes (Michela Luciani, 2022).

Focusing on taking care of yourself physically, spiritually, and emotionally by prioritizing your needs and desires is the shortest way to get in sync with your dark feminine energy.

You can do countless things to implement self-care; here are some ideas that worked for many of my clients:

- **Take care of your body:** I know it may seem trivial, but eating regularly and in the right way, sleeping the correct hours, and doing physical activity help your body and mind. When our body has found balance, our mind can unleash all its potential.

- **Practice self-expression:** Many activities can activate your creative side and express your emotions. In addition to enriching you as a person, they can help you connect with your inner self. For example, dancing or creating music are great passions to pursue. In my case, journaling helped me open up about myself.

- **Practice self-reflection:** To be self-confident, you must first know yourself thoroughly. Allocating time throughout the day to introspect and work on gaining greater awareness of your thoughts and feelings is essential for tapping into both the light and dark feminine energy. If you don't know where to start, don't worry, I'll introduce you to some basic self-reflection techniques you can use daily.

- **Nurture relationships:** Surrounding yourself with a few valuable people is essential. A circle of friends and relatives that support you in your everyday life, regardless of your choices, is vital for self-esteem. In this case, self-care is not about us but our relationships with these people. Finding time to be with them and share moments of our lives can give us that extra security to truly bring out what we have inside.

- **Practice self-compassion:** One of the main obstacles to connecting with your dark feminine energy is self-criticism and negative self-talk. Unfortunately, we are our worst critics, and these self-destructive practices make it challenging to acquire the confidence we need to tap into the hidden side of our personality freely. If you don't know where to start, don't worry; in this chapter, I'll show you several techniques to help you practice self-compassion and assume a more positive attitude towards yourself.

Before starting with the techniques of self-reflection and self-compassion, I would like to emphasize one point. Self-care is a personal and individual practice, and what works for one person may not work for another.

In this chapter, I provide suggestions and methods that work for the most varied types of people. But, of course, hardly one person will use them all, and some will not be effective for you. Before starting, I suggest taking a few minutes to figure out what you really need.

For example, if you are an already extremely positive woman and don't practice excessive self-criticism, you may not need self-compassion techniques. On the other hand, if you are a woman used to introspection and have experience with meditation, further self-reflection techniques could be a waste of your time. In short, feel free to skip parts of this book that you think don't apply to you. This volume is meant to help you manifest your dark feminine energy, but you will find your way to do it.

Also, remember that self-care must be sustainable and integrated into your life regularly. It's no use trying 10 different things for a week, and then realizing you're doing too much. Self-care doesn't have to become a job.

Instead, focus only on the suggestions you find most interesting and see if they are helpful for you. Then, occasionally, you can introduce something new and remove something that didn't work or that you think you no longer need.

SELF-REFLECTION IN PRACTICE

These techniques will help you learn who you are and uncover hidden sides of your personality. For many women, they are, therefore, a great way to get in touch with their dark feminine. Also, understanding yourself is one of the most important things for mental wellbeing. For these reasons, I suggest taking 10 minutes a day to focus on self-reflection activity. Ensure that in your self-reflection time, you are alone in a quiet environment without distractions.

I will share some questions to guide you during your sessions. They will help you focus on the right things and get the best results. Remember that you are asking these questions to your subconscious; it is not like running a job interview. Instead, you are trying to engage the deeper layers of your mind for an answer. For this reason, an honest answer might not come immediately. Instead, you might have to dig into your subconscious, asking the same question multiple times until you feel you have reached the honest answer. Take your time, and don't be happy with the first answer your brain gives you; this is often just a reflective habit but not the truth you seek. Many women need multiple sessions per question to engage the deepest level of their subconscious. This is normal and a journey every person takes at their own pace.

One last piece of advice, in my experience, the questions that cause the most emotional tension have an answer that contains more insights than the others.

In sterquiliniis invenitur—in filth it will be found.

This alchemical phrase from the Middle Ages loosely translates to: "What you need most is where you least want to look." Naturally, you will be tempted to "run-away" and accept one of the first answers you get. Force yourself to dig deeper instead, and you will find what you need most.

Here is the first question you should ask yourself:

"What do I want?"

To become who you want to be, you must understand what you want. I'm not talking about what you want in three months or a year, but what you want in life.

This question may seem trivial, but a world is hidden behind it. Especially for young women, you may find that what you do in your life isn't what you want; it is what other people want for you. Many women seek other people's approval; others are afraid to take risks and decide to play it safe.

When I asked myself this question, I remember figuring out what I wanted took me some time. But the most important thing I realized in answering this question was that I was going in the wrong direction. My actions would never get me where I wanted to be.

Once you know your deepest desires, you acquire an entirely different perspective. Your scale of values suddenly changes; things that previously seemed all-important are not so relevant anymore. For instance, I never really wanted to make a career in a multinational corporation, and once I realized that, some things that pained me at work lost all power over me. Ironically, I began performing better once I started caring less and gained more confidence through the introspection work I'd completed. However, although I was starting to get appreciated at that point, my long-term plan had changed, and I quit a few months later.

Second question:

"What am I avoiding?"

This question has a deeper meaning than "I avoid taking out the trash." With this question, you want to identify your uncertainties and what you fear and therefore avoid. Our fears guide us in everyday life, direct our actions, influence our thoughts, and prevent us from using our full potential. Thus, to connect with our dark feminine energy, we must identify our fears in our subconscious.

Every woman has many fears, and being aware of what you are avoiding will be the first step in taking control of them. By bringing conscious attention to your worries, they will lessen in degree; you will be able to understand them better, so you can confront them more effectively.

Third question:

"What am I most grateful for in my life?"

Positivity and negativity are always part of our life, from childhood to adulthood.

Although individuals vary in how optimistic they are about the future, one assumption that researchers make is that optimism is sensitive to changes in life events and circumstances.

[...]Optimism is an individual attribute that is ~25% heritable but can also be learned and shaped by social influences (Chopik, 2020).

Sometimes our brain has an implicit negativity bias, leading us to see things from a more pessimistic point of view. Of course, this doesn't apply to everyone, but it is true for most people. An example of this bias is when we focus only on what we don't have and what others have. To a certain degree, this can be a motivating stimulus to do better and achieve one's goals, but it can also become a problem. It's one thing to be motivated to achieve a particular purpose; it's another thing to feel miserable.

Observing the world through these lenses makes us continually highlight all our shortcomings and does not make us give enough weight to what we have built in our lives.

With this question, we want to build a new mental habit. We want to change this mechanism that leads us to belittle our achievements. Instead, we want to learn to recognize and celebrate our successes, and finally give them the importance they deserve.

Changing how we see things doesn't happen overnight, but it all starts with this simple question: "What am I most grateful for in my life?"

As with the other questions, your mind initially gives you pre-packaged answers. Yet, they are the ones you use in your everyday life. Your job will be to dig deep to find the real answers that mean something, the ones that make you emotional.

Fourth question:

"What are my biggest strengths and flaws?"

This question can help you discover sides of yourself that you don't appreciate enough. For example, many women have low self-esteem, and some even go as far as self-loathing.

I'm not ashamed to say that I didn't like myself in my youth before starting my self-reflection journey. Focusing mainly on my flaws was the norm, leading me to lose self-confidence and affecting my ability to relate to others.

Gaining a conscious awareness of your strengths that balances out your flaws is vital in knowing yourself and being able to channel sides of your personality that you didn't think existed.

There is a substantial difference between pretending to be a femme fatale and feeling like a femme fatale. Playing a part is easy, but being one requires a deep knowledge of what you have inside. You have to learn your limitations and also your strengths, so you can use them.

Remember that for every strength, there is a shadow weakness; you can't have one without the other. So, if you see yourself as fundamentally flawed, then you probably need to look at the bigger picture. It is impossible to have all the weaknesses we so easily find in ourselves without having the strengths associated with them.

As usual, this doesn't come free. You must do introspection work to understand your inherent positive or creative qualities. If you think about it, this is very similar to the yin-yang concept. Weaknesses and strengths are opposite interconnected forces; it is up to you to discover them. Take your time, ask yourself these questions, and I promise you will find them.

SELF-COMPASSION IN PRACTICE

In this section, I'll show you different ways to practice self-compassion.

Let's start with the **self-compassion break** technique. This approach consists of guided meditation to help you focus on your problems, forgive yourself, and let them go. This is a way to let go of what weighs down your mind, undermines your self-confidence, and could be an obstacle to accessing your dark feminine energy.

I want to teach you to bring a little tenderness and love to yourself, especially if you find yourself in a moment of difficulty.

Guided meditation: Think of a situation where you need care and love. It could be a situation where you feel inadequate or think you've made a mistake. You may focus on something you don't like or find difficult. Something in your life that isn't working out how you want it.

Mentally try to enter this situation; think about how it made you feel or still makes you feel. Feel the discomfort in your body, reviving what makes you feel suffering.

When you believe you are in contact with these negative feelings, it is time to call into play the three elements of self-compassion.

Let's start with **mindfulness**. This is simply being present in the moment and validating the pain. I want you to learn to communicate with yourself and recognize pain for this part of the exercise. First, tell yourself, "It's tough to think about this situation and feel the feelings it awakens in me." Then, give yourself a few seconds to accept that this is a moment of pain in which you feel uncomfortable.

Now, it's time to start thinking about your humanity. There is nothing wrong with feeling this way; many other people have the same problems and feelings. It's all part of being human and living in this world; your problems are similar to others, but at the same time, unique; we are all connected. So, allow yourself to feel your **connectedness** to others in your own imperfections.

As a last step, we want to bring some **kindness** into play. One way to do this is with a specific breathing technique and physical touch.

Let's start with breathing, repeat the following steps until you feel calm and focused:

- **Step 1:** Inhale for four seconds through your nose.
- **Step 2:** Hold your breath for two seconds.
- **Step 3:** Exhale through the nose for six seconds.
- **Step 4:** Take a short pause of one second before inhaling again.

As you focus on breathing, start slowly caressing your belly or face. Feel the warmth of your hands on your skin and let yourself be carried away by the feeling of peace.

When you feel ready, try saying something kind to yourself. It could be a message of acceptance or forgiveness. For example, you could tell yourself something like "It is okay to be imperfect" or a supportive message such as "I'm here for you; I won't abandon you." Think about what you need most, what you want to hear, and say it.

Repeat it a few times, focus on what it means to you, on the positive feelings it awakens in you, and slowly try to let go of that situation that made you suffer.

Take the time you need and finish the session when you want. Remember, you are in control. When you feel ready, return to the real world with more love for yourself and greater awareness.

Another technique you could use is called **self-soothing**. This technique is based on participation in activities that can give you positive feelings and make you feel loved. These activities are very subjective and therefore vary from woman to woman.

The basic idea is that everyone has to experiment to find suitable activities that can convey sensations of care and kindness toward themselves.

These activities don't have to be anything special; eating pizza with a friend, going to your favorite restaurant, going for a walk, or indulging in a few hours at the spa can be perfect for taking care of yourself.

If you don't want to leave the house, even sipping a good glass of wine while reading a book or listening to music can be considered a self-soothing activity. The important thing is that it conveys feelings of care and kindness towards yourself.

These activities aim to make your mind realize that you deserve to feel good and fight that little voice we all have in our heads that tends to attack us.

Remember that this is not about pursuing a hobby or taking a break. The fundamental thing is that these activities, whatever they are, make you feel truly pampered and appreciated.

In my case, my go-to self-soothing activity is gardening. I love the contact with nature, the feeling of taking care of something alive, the slowness and repetitiveness of the movements, and the sun on the skin can calm me down and make me feel loved and at peace with myself.

Find the activity that gives you these sensations and practice it for at least 30 minutes weekly. I assure you that it will slowly change your approach to the world if done with awareness.

CHAPTER 5

You Come First

There is no limit to what we, as women, can accomplish.
—Michelle Obama

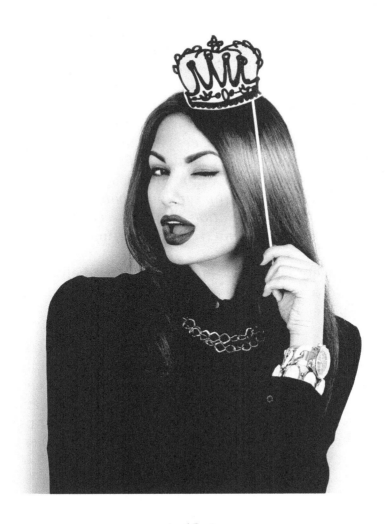

Putting yourself first is an essential aspect of self-care and self-love, which are pillars that allow you to find the right balance and access your dark feminine energy. A femme fatale always puts herself first.

Some might call "putting yourself first" as "being selfish," but is this actually a bad thing?

> *Selfishness is often regarded as an undesirable or even immoral characteristic, whereas altruism is typically considered universally desirable and virtuous. However, human history as well as the works of humanistic and psychodynamic psychologists point to a more complex picture: not all selfishness is necessarily bad, and not all altruism is necessarily good.[...] In his 1939 essay "Selfishness and Self-Love," Erich Fromm opened by declaring that "Modern culture is pervaded by a taboo on selfishness. It teaches that to be selfish is sinful and that to love others is virtuous." In his essay, Fromm argues that this cultural taboo has had the unfortunate consequence of making people feel guilty to show themselves healthy self-love, which he defines as the passionate affirmation and respect for one's own happiness, growth, and freedom* (Kaufman, 2020).

Modern society is founded on the idea that helping others is good, but have you ever stopped considering whether this is actually implemented?

Famous people are great at raising money for a charitable cause if it helps them improve their public relations. Wealthy people are committed to cleaning up the seas that their own companies pollute. Giant corporations exploit other continents and populations to produce the objects we use daily at meager prices. Of course, there are exceptions, but altruism and capitalism generally do not work well together.

Why, then, should you feel guilty prioritizing yourself compared to others? You will not hurt anyone if you treat yourself to a spa day, or if, instead of silently following the group's choices, you choose which movie to see on your night off.

On top of that, research has shown that by practicing kindness to yourself, you experience greater levels of happiness (Rowland, 2018).

In this chapter, I, therefore, want to answer the following questions:

- What does it mean to put yourself first?
- How can you put yourself first?

Putting yourself first means not ignoring your needs or sacrificing your dreams in favor of others. This does not necessarily imply being selfish in a negative sense; when you care for your own physical, emotional, and mental wellbeing, you are better set up to take care of others, too.

Putting yourself first means you have time to do self-care, connect with your body, practice tantra, and all the other activities that might help you channel your dark feminine energy.

Putting your actual needs, self-respect, and integrity first is just one aspect of "you come first;" on the other hand, it is essential not to let others walk over you.

From my experience, this second part is the one I have always found more challenging. Especially from a very young age being able to relate to others and put my needs in front of those of other people has never been easy. However, luckily with practice, you get better!

There are several handy techniques to keep others from walking over you.

SET BOUNDARIES

Boundaries are delineations where another person ends, and you begin. It is like having a contract with another person that regulates how you will behave in your relationship.

When a person struggles to be assertive, this often happens because there are no firm boundaries, and others feel entitled to invade spaces they should not.

Boundaries are a primary tool for putting yourself first.

Assertiveness, if you remember, is one of the characteristics of dark feminine. Therefore, setting boundaries helps create time for yourself and act like a dark feminine. Boundaries are not like insurmountable walls, but they help to define what you will and won't tolerate; in short, they allow you to be in charge of your life.

You can set boundaries around:

- time
- personal space
- sexuality
- material possessions
- finances
- morals and ethics

Your boundaries can be set in different ways with:

- family
- friends
- strangers
- partner
- coworkers

The first step in defining your boundaries is to visualize your limits. For this exercise, I advise you to use a notebook; this will help you translate the abstract boundaries that until now have lived only in your mind into concrete and applicable rules.

First, ask yourself the following questions and write the answers in your notebook or here, if you prefer:

What is my primary source of stress or discomfort?

_____

What excites me every day and makes me happy?

_____

What quenches my enthusiasm?

_____

What makes me unhappy?

_____

What parts of my life suck up all my energy?

_____

What makes me feel safe and supported?

_____

After answering these questions, you should start to have an initial clarity on your limits; in this second part of the exercise, we'll define them even better. Take a page from your notebook and draw a circle in the center of the page. Make the circle cover about half the page. If you prefer, you can use the space provided on page 49.

Inside the circle, write everything that makes you feel safe and stress-free.

Outside the circle, write down anything that bothers you, stresses you out, or makes your life physically or emotionally challenging.

Here is an example of my circle:

My friend Samantha constantly dumping her relationship problems on me

Working after-hours instead of prioritizing my needs

My cat Lilly

Dancing, Jogging

Walking in the park

Shopping with my sister and mother

Watching Netflix on the couch with a glass of wine

Singing at the Karaoke

Cooking with my partner

Hugs from my partner

Play with my nephew

My mother telling me to have babies

People on the train touching me

Worry about the impression that I leave on people

My partner listening to music without headphones

Here some space for you to complete your circle:

When your circle is complete, you will have a graphical representation of your limits. The next step is translating everything outside your circle into a boundary you can communicate to your friends, family, etc.

Retake your notebook and define boundaries to help prevent or remove all elements outside your circle. For example, if outside the circle, you have written something like: "people in a bar touching me without asking permission." You could translate this limit into a personal space boundary to communicate to strangers: "I don't feel comfortable being touched by anyone. If you don't intend to respect my space, I will leave."

This is just a basic example; how you decide to communicate your boundaries could change from situation to situation. But the idea is always the same: take your limits and look for a way to communicate them to the people you want to interact with. Remember that you want to be as clear and firm as possible. It doesn't need to be a long sentence; a few words are usually enough to set the tone for future interactions.

Let me give you another example. Imagine that you wrote something outside your circle, like "Supporting friends emotionally when I am having an emotionally difficult time."

You can translate your limit into the following boundary and communicate it to your friend: "I'm sorry you're having a hard time; unfortunately, I'm having a hard time too, and I don't have the emotional bandwidth to have this discussion at the moment."

Proceed now to translate all your limits into boundaries you can easily communicate; in the following paragraphs, we will learn how to defend them from other people's "attacks."

LEARN TO SAY NO

The best way to defend your boundaries is to learn to say "no" when needed. Although it may sound simple to some, it is a complex task for many women.

The reasons why this is challenging vary significantly from woman to woman, but the following are, in my experience, the most common reasons:

- feeling guilty or obligated
- being afraid that people will think poorly of you, or you'll disappoint them
- being a people pleaser
- avoiding conflicts
- saying "yes" to everything is a habit
- be polite or be seen as a nice person
- fear of missing out (FOMO)

Do any of these reasons sound familiar to you? You'll be surprised how many people the above list resonates with. Saying "no" is not a joke; for some, it is like climbing a high mountain. However, here are some tips for defending your boundaries by saying fewer yeses.

Don't explain: When you refuse something, the politest thing to do seems to invent a plausible excuse. The problem is that a highly determined person could find a way around your excuse, leaving you practically forced to accept. So, instead of coming up with a reason, thank them for the offer, tell them you can't accept it, and offer no further explanation. It's not about being rude; you can be polite even without providing different answers by enriching your refusal with things like "I'm sorry I can't do this" or similar.

Rehearse your no: Rejecting something via email or text is more straightforward than doing it in person. However, when you have to decline in person, the best thing you can do if you don't feel comfortable declining an offer is to practice saying "no." For example, if you know a friend will invite you to a concert you do not want to attend, prepare your refusal strategy before going out.

Practice being natural and polite in turning down the offer in front of the mirror, so when it's time to say "no" for real, you'll know how to do it.

Use "later": Sometimes saying "no" is extremely complicated, while saying "later" is relatively simple. If you're in a situation where you can't turn down something you don't want to do, start buying time by putting off the problem. Simple phrases like "let me get back to you" or "let me check my schedule and get back to you later" can reduce the momentary pressure to say yes and decide the best way to decline.

Offer an alternative: In some cases, you want to say no but at the same time maintain a good relationship with the person who is asking you to do something. Offering an alternative, in this case, can help maintain good relations. For example: "Apologies, I won't be able to do X, but let me introduce you to my friend Marissa; she is very skilled in X, and I'm sure she will be able to help."

Use a non-verbal "no": Sixty to ninety-five percent of communication is non-verbal (Crane, 2010). Sometimes, if your conversational partner is paying enough attention, refusing a proposal explicitly will not be necessary; your body will speak for you. To communicate a firm no with your body, try rotating your torso, so you are not face-to-face with the person. Cross your arms to assume a defensive stance. Point your feet as if you are about to walk away from the discussion at any moment. This is usually enough to convey a resounding non-verbal "no."

It may not be necessary to use all of these non-verbal cues si-multaneously; even one may be enough to convey the message. Do not worry if you are unfamiliar with body language; given the power of non-verbal communication, I have dedicated a separate chapter to go deeper into this topic.

Chapter 6
Indulge Yourself

*It took me quite a long time to develop a voice, and now
that I have it, I am not going to be silent.*
—Madeleine Albright

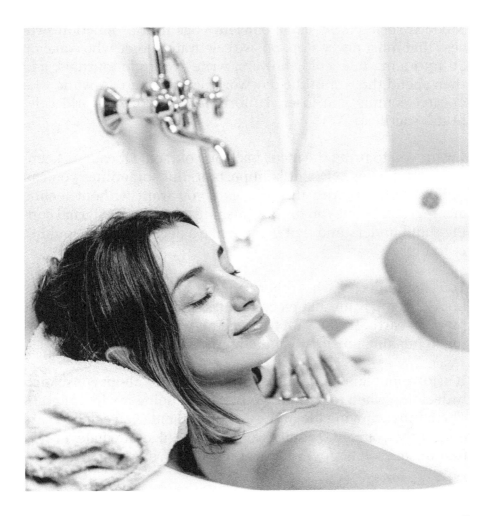

earning to indulge yourself without shame or guilt is a powerful way to channel our dark feminine energy. For example, how often have you said to yourself, "I can't have that piece of chocolate because..." or felt guilty because you did not go to the gym, slept more in the morning, or instead of doing something as a priority, spent the afternoon watching Netflix?

It's like having a conflict in our bodies. Two energies tell us to do two opposite things. If we follow what one tells us, we are good girls. If we follow what the other tells us, we are bad girls.

Modern society sees us as efficient cogs in a production process that must never stop. So, we celebrate people who wake up at 4:30 a.m., take cold showers, write gratitude journals, and then spend the rest of the day working for others. Anyone who doesn't comply is a loser. Unfortunately, today's world celebrates sacrifice.

I want you to bring the focus back on yourself. Of course, keeping fit and being efficient is important, but sometimes you can indulge yourself with the chocolate you want without feeling any regrets. I want you to start pushing away these internal conflicts and understand that if you make a decision, you shouldn't regret it.

You shouldn't care what other people, or the world say, it is your life. So, if you want that piece of chocolate, eat it like it's the last piece on earth. If you want to spend an hour in a hot bath listening to relaxing music by candlelight, go for it.

It's not about ignoring your commitments. It's about consciously deciding when to pamper yourself and doing it without guilt. Then, fully enjoying life in those few moments you can dedicate entirely to yourself. Indulge yourself. Indulge in whatever it is that makes you happy; whatever it is that brings you joy.

START PRACTICING TANTRA DAILY

Some may consider tantra solely as a sexual practice, but there is much more. Tantra is an ancient life-embracing philosophy that originated in India in the 6th century. It teaches that everything is sacred, including sensuality.

In tantric vision, the world is animated by divine feminine energy. Shakti is one of the principal deities and contrasts with the time's female representations. Indeed, Shakti is sensual and powerful.

Why do I recommend practicing tantra? Because tantra teaches us to connect our body with our spirit. It is a path that leads to knowing ourselves through pleasure. It's not a fundamental step to unveil our femme fatale. However, it's an excellent help to discover some attributes of dark feminine energy, including the pursuit of pleasure. When practiced correctly, I trust that tantra can help you identify your dark feminine energy, as it did with many other women and me.

Given the limited space of this book, I will not approach tantra from a philosophical point of view. Instead, I will limit myself to practical exercises to help you connect with your dark feminine energy.

Tantra can be trivialized as "find pleasure in all things," and I want you to learn to do that. According to a study conducted in 2015 (Berridge):

> *In a sense, pleasure can be thought of as evolution's boldest trick, serving to motivate an individual to pursue rewards necessary for fitness, career, success[...] An important starting point for understanding the underlying circuitry [in our brain] is to recognize that rewards involve a composite of several psychological components: liking[...], wanting[...], and learning[...].*

One of the traits of a woman in tune with her dark feminine energy is that she can take pleasure for herself. So, you can start doing it through small things at your own pace, stimulating your mind with unusual sensations, while tapping into your dark feminine energy.

This will train your body to become familiar with the feeling of pleasure, and thanks to how our brain works, it will push you to create automatisms to always seek this sensation more.

Explaining how to do it is not straightforward, but the idea is to slow down, feel yourself, and feel pleasure in your actions. For example, the next time you eat something, do not rush it. Instead, savor every bite, and appreciate the range of flavors. Forget about your commitments for a moment, and if you are eating a dessert, take a spoonful and let it melt in your mouth.

You must learn to find pleasure and take it for yourself. For example, sometimes eating can be like making love; you want to reward your brain with that sweet sensation.

There are many things you can try to get in touch with all your senses. For example, spoil yourself with a new silk nightgown or new sheets and feel how they caress you. Feel the silk on your skin.

Go to the park and enjoy the spring sun on your body while reading a good book on the grass.

Don't do the usual five-minute shower. Instead of a quick scrub, slow down, caress your body, enjoy the touch of your hands, use scented soaps to stimulate your sense of smell, and maybe spoil yourself with some new soft towels. It is not just about enjoying the sensations but also about realizing that you deserve to be pampered and making your brain learn that pleasure is not something to escape from. Learn to enjoy with all your senses.

And there's more. Tantra is a practice that involves sexual acts. You need total synchronicity and collaboration with your partner to practice it correctly. I won't explore it further because it's a long and complex topic, and the space in this book is strictly limited to our dark feminine energy. However, if I have piqued your curiosity, I invite you to deepen it starting with the book by Samantha Mandala, *Tantric Sex Guide for Couples*.

CHAPTER 7

Connect With Your Body and Sexuality

We need to reshape our own perception of how we view ourselves.
We have to step up as women and take the lead.
—Beyoncé

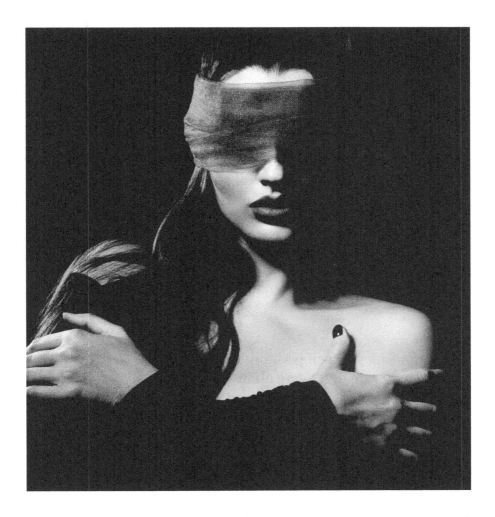

ast but not least, one powerful way to tap into your dark feminine energy is to do it from its most sensual side. Sensuality and femme fatale have always gone hand in hand in the collective imagination. Although the dark feminine energy is not limited to this, the sensual sphere certainly plays a role of primary importance.

Sensuality is a personal and subjective experience; there is no instruction manual or good and evil. Therefore, what makes me happy may not be sensually fulfilling for another woman and vice versa. For this reason, in this part of the book, it isn't easy to give advice that applies to all readers, so you may disagree with some of the suggested techniques or not find them particularly interesting. But one thing applies to all women; not everyone remembers it, even if it is trivial:

It's important to honor your desires and boundaries and not compare yourself to others.

If there are things you don't feel comfortable doing, don't do them. Sensuality is personal, and you must experience it as you wish. Part of being a femme fatale is knowing precisely what you want and don't, but this only develops with experience.

If you are a young woman or you are still discovering your sensuality, knowing precisely what you want may not be clear. In addition, various factors could push you out of your comfort zone for the wrong reasons:

• peer pressure
• comparing yourself with others
• partners who don't care about you enough
• the desire to please someone and make them happy

To embrace your inner dark feminine, one of the first steps is that you should not feel obligated to try things you're not sure about, and you should feel free to experience what you're curious about regardless of other people's judgment.

Sensuality is a space where any woman must be free to express herself as she wishes, without external influences and pressures.

KNOW WHAT YOU LIKE

Throughout this book, I have repeated more than once that a woman in tune with her dark feminine energy knows how to take pleasure for herself and satisfy her needs. Of course, this is true in every field of life, even in bed. But how can you get what you want if you don't know everything you like?

Part of becoming a femme fatale is introspection and self-exploration to figure out what you want and how you want it. Self-exploration is a theme that will frequently recur, given that it has multiple benefits, not just that of helping you understand what you like. It can also be a means to connect with your sexual energy, relax, or reduce performance anxiety. It is a natural way to boost your confidence and show a different side of you to your partner.

By self-exploration, in this specific context, I mean spending time alone exploring your body and learning what feels pleasurable or exciting. If you don't know where to start or you have never spent much time thinking about it, here are some ideas for practicing self-exploration:

- Run your fingernails lightly over your scalp, paying particular attention to the areas above the neck and behind the ears.

- Stimulate your navel by tracing circular movements with your fingertips descending progressively toward the genitals.

- Run your fingertips slowly along the inner arm to the armpit.

- Caress the inner thigh with slow and light movements.

- Try massaging the bottom of your feet, testing different levels of pressure.

- See how other areas of your body react to the light stimulation of a feather.

- Massage your body with oil.

- Play with your nipples to see how they react to touch.

- Play with your clitoris, exploring different levels of pressure.

- Play with your clitoris, exploring different motions.

- Play with a dildo, giving an internal vaginal massage.

These are just a few examples, but feel free to try whatever you think might be interesting, there is no limit to your creativity.

I also advise you to write down the sensations you experienced for each technique you wanted to experiment with. Then, after a few self-exploration sessions, it will be easier to have an objective picture of what you actually like.

STOP SHAMING YOUR BODY!

Our body is an essential vessel of sexual energy, which is directly connected to our inner dark feminine. However, many women find it challenging to be in tune with their bodies and accept themselves. As a result, many of them set unattainable standards or are ruthless when judging themselves. For this reason, it becomes almost impossible for some people to feel sensual and at ease in their bodies.

Once again, I return to the concept of self-care and practicing self-compassion; everything starts from there. If we don't love ourselves, we cannot love our bodies, making us insecure.

Sensuality is the least of our thoughts in this situation of reduced self-confidence since we find it hard even to look in the mirror without judging ourselves.

The solution is simple, and it is called **self-love**.

I know self-love is overused, and for some of us, it doesn't matter how many pleasant things we say about ourselves; it just doesn't feel genuine. I get it; I've been there.

If you don't feel authentic when you practice self-compassion, you can try practicing **body neutrality**. In my experience, it works for many women, myself included.

Body neutrality can slowly lead us to accept our body for what it is. Of course, it takes time and patience, like all things in the world, but trying doesn't hurt!

With body neutrality, I want you to learn not to actively shame your body, bringing you one step closer to connecting with your sensual energy and your inner dark feminine.

Body neutrality is just a fancy name for a straightforward, and at the same time, challenging-to-master practice. Everything starts with this simple rule:

You no longer want to say or think anything negative about your body.

But, at the same time, you don't need to keep telling yourself positive things you might not believe. Put simply; you should actively stop telling yourself negative things.

It may sound strange, but one of the tricks that help me apply body neutrality is mentally taking a step back from the current situation and thinking about dogs. Yes, dogs, I know, I'm a strange person! I love dogs; they come in all breeds and sizes and are always joyful and adorable. If I were a dog, I would probably feel like a bulldog: chubby, lazy, and cute.

If you think about it, we set beauty standards for humans that are almost impossible to achieve, but every dog is the cutest thing in the world. When I think about it, I don't feel like telling myself I have the most toned butt in the world, but it makes me smile, and I don't feel like diminishing my body anymore. I know it sounds stupid, but it works for me!

There is no sure-fire recipe for practicing body neutrality; you must find something that blocks your negative thoughts and bring it to mind when needed. It can be anything if it prevents you from actively shaming your body. I remember a client of mine loved flowers and used a vivid image of an orchid to stop negative thoughts.

An alternative approach to stop body shaming yourself is giving your body the pleasure it deserves. You can do it in various ways, by touching yourself, using scented oils, relaxing baths, and caring for your hair and nails. The idea is to experience pleasurable sensations with all five senses while caring for your body. This shifts your mind from "how my body looks" to "how my body feels." As a result, your mind will leave behind negative feelings in search of further pleasure. As you can see, we circled back to indulging ourselves and practicing tantra. It is all linked.

FOCUS ON PLEASURE, NOT JUST PERFORMANCE

Have you ever felt not connected with your sensuality and your body or insecure during the sexual act? Having a lack of sexual confidence is quite common in women of all ages; this can happen for various reasons and depends a lot on the context and previous experiences. For example, if you find yourself thinking a lot about sexual performance, perhaps worrying more about how your partner sees you than living in the moment, this may be keeping you from connecting with your senses.

If what I wrote sounds familiar, the rest of this section may help. The lack of sensual confidence is like a wall we build in front of us. This mighty obstacle is difficult to break, and it prevents us from really connecting with our senses and fully experiencing the moment with our partner. It's hard to feel pleasure when you're focused on how the performance is going and not on the feelings you're experiencing.

One thing to remember is that, in many cases, this wall has no sense of existing. So, it is very likely that our partner is not judging you in the moments of intimacy you spend together, and they are simply enjoying being with you.

Many coaches would tell you, "relax and enjoy it," but this is not a solution, is it?

No magic wand can suddenly change your mental attitude and allow you to experience sensuality in a freer and more relaxed way. If you are stressed about sexual performance, you will continue to be stressed even after hearing, "you should relax." However, here are some tips and tricks you can apply to help you focus more on the pleasure and less on the performance.

- **Focus on the touch:** Touch is one of the most stimulated senses during sex and is undoubtedly the most involved. The next time you make love to your partner, focus solely on the sensation it causes to have his hands on your body and how you feel when it is touched. Don't think about the act of penetration. Instead, caress each other and bring your bodies into contact as much as possible. Try to abandon yourself to the sense of touch and live it as a meditation exercise to reconnect with yourself.

- **Stress is your enemy:** Stress is a factor that can impact our sexual performance and how we experience sensuality in general. This problem manifests itself more in men with the inability to get an erection, but it can also occur in a different form in women. Stress can make us approach sex the wrong way and interfere with the sensations we experience.

Women in the high-stress group have no psychological arousal,[...] have higher levels of cortisol, and report less focus[...] (Hamilton, 2013).

A simple way to reduce stress is to exercise regularly. For example, a 20–30-minute exercise routine a few times a week can boost overall wellbeing and reduce stress levels, which may be helpful.

- **Take some time with yourself:** One way to reduce performance anxiety is to allocate some time to masturbate regularly. I'm not talking about a few minutes spent with a vibrator but a good half hour exploring your body, enjoying your touch, and connecting with more powerful orgasmic sensations. You want to spend time massaging your body and feeling your fingers on your skin. The idea is to treat self-pleasure like a meditation session, with no shame, awareness that you deserve pleasure, and can take your time and pace to get it. This is a way to train your body and mind to feel powerful sensations.

- **Communicate with your partner:** Once you realize what you like through self-pleasure sessions, it will be easier to speak with your partner about how you want things done, naming your needs. If you believe you deserve pleasure, everything will begin to line up. You can start to say, "I would like to do it like this," instead of tolerating receiving pleasure in a way that doesn't work for you.

Trust me, once you realize how to name your needs and prioritize them, it will change your world entirely. You will start to align the things you desire with the sensations you are feeling in the moment, and you will take pleasure for yourself.

A short personal note, my family has always been very old-fashioned, and I can say that I started to discover sensuality late compared to some of my peers. This isn't necessarily bad, but I felt stressed in my first relationships with my partners due to a lack of experience.

If there's one thing that really helped me out of all the advice in this section, it was starting to take self-exploration sessions seriously. An opportunity to learn more about my body, not to limit myself to a simple, quick orgasm, but to create the mood, relax, and take all the time and pleasure I deserve.

CHALLENGE YOUR NEGATIVE BELIEFS ABOUT SEX

As I said, my family was quite old-fashioned, and my parents never addressed the topic of sexuality openly with my brothers or me. At school, sex education was limited, in my case, to lots of laughs, learning how to use contraceptives, and avoiding getting pregnant at all costs. In church, of course, discussing sex was taboo, and with friends, it was more giggles than anything else.

If you have had a similar experience growing up, this could have created implicit limitations to your sensuality; in extreme cases, it even leads to becoming sex-negative or sexually repressed.

I don't want to send the wrong message, and I want to clarify this point as much as possible.

Sexual repression is not asexuality, genuine disinterest in experimenting with sexual practices, or having a limited sexual experience.

Sexual repression is a state in which a person is prevented from expressing their own sexuality. Sexual repression is often associated with feelings of guilt or shame associated with sexual impulses (Sexual_repression, n.d.).

External and internal factors cause sexual repression; it is basically the sum of how you grew up and feel. Sexual repression is not as common as you might think and having strict parents doesn't automatically cause it, despite what some influencers on TikTok may say.

As a woman, it's much more likely that you haven't fully explored your sensuality due to some mental barriers.

In this part, I will cover the most common sex stereotypes and negative beliefs that may or may not affect your sexual life.

Sex is all about him: Have you ever lived in a relationship where your partner always takes the initiative, even when you are not in the mood? He always wants to touch you, grab you, and when you have sex with him, it is always about his pleasure, his orgasms. Does this sound familiar?

Unfortunately, many women tend to indulge their partner's wishes too much, to the detriment of their own. The result is highly counterproductive because if on the one hand, they believe they are doing him a favor, on the other, they turn off their sensuality, and what should be a magical moment becomes little more than a formality to be dealt with quickly. It's like turning off your imagination and creativity and taking the passenger seat in the sexual act.

If it resonates with you, you must understand sex is a two-way street where you both work for the goal of pleasure with an ultimate connection. So, don't be afraid to take what is yours, and don't subordinate your needs to anyone else's.

Trust me when I say that you can both be happy and satisfied. Switching from a passive to an active role in your relationship is a great way to connect with your dark feminine energy. I'm sure your partner will be pleasantly surprised by your newfound initiative and confidence.

If I share my desires and needs, I will be judged: Regardless of how common or exotic your desires are, not sharing them is a lose-lose situation for you and your partner.

The thing is that your partner has no way of knowing what you desire, need, or want during sex unless you show or tell them. If you say nothing, then nothing will change. You may be judged if you say something, but that's not your problem. If someone judges you for what you like or want to experience in bed, they are probably not the right person for you, and it is not worth wasting your time with them.

I want to give you the example of a client of mine, whom we will call Janine. She had been in a stable relationship for a few years and was happy, but she felt something was missing.

During one of our chats, Janine explained that she wanted to experiment with bondage on her partner. She had always been intrigued by this practice and would have liked to try it sometime to fulfill her fantasies. However, her relationship had well-defined dynamics, her partner had always taken an active role, and she didn't feel at ease discussing these practices with him.

Flash forwards a couple of weeks, and with some moral support and convincing, Janine decides to open up to her partner. The discussion with him wasn't challenging like she expected.

In our next chat, she told me they tried bondage several times, and he was enthusiastic about trying something new. Unfortunately, she also told me that she had imagined the whole experience differently; perhaps it was one of those things we idealize and think exciting, but it didn't click for them when they tried. However, she was happy to have discussed it with her partner. One thing less on her bucket list.

In this story, there is a happy ending, but let's try now to think what would have happened if Janine's partner had rejected her requests or, even worse, had judged her for her needs and desires. Janine would have been faced with a necessary reality. Right or wrong, her partner was unwilling to indulge in her wishes. It would have been up to her to decide how much of a deal-breaker this was for their relationship and how to act. Better to be honest than to live with unexpressed desires.

Religious, sexual shame: In the USA, we are reaping the benefits of decades of religiously influenced sex education. Schools teach students about abstinence instead of preparing them for sexual intercourse. Along with abstinence-only education came the concept of "purity" and the morally based belief that remaining pure from sexuality until marriage was a good, moral, and desired choice (D., 2017).

On top of it, Christianity considers sex solely and exclusively as a reproductive method. All these factors led to a highly unprepared generation being able to openly connect with their sexuality.

If this resonates with you and, like many others, you have been involved in one of these purity movements that could have impacted your natural sexual development, know that there are ways to experience unrestrained sensuality without abandoning your religious beliefs.

The topic is vast, and a separate book would be needed to cover it entirely; for this reason, I recommend Tina Schermer's book Sex, God & the Conservative Church. It is a great read and helped many people overcome church-induced sexual shame.

Sexuality is not learned! Nothing is more false; sexuality is something you master over time, and everyone can be great lovers. Sexuality is 90% practical and 10% creative. Especially in women, sexual fulfillment comes with time. This is to say that, even if you don't consider yourself the best lover in the world, honing your skills as a seductress is mainly about practice. Some people may be predisposed to be fiery lovers, but experience pays off.

If my partner didn't have an orgasm, it didn't go well!
I've had this discussion many times with various clients, and I always respond similarly. It's not just your responsibility that your partner has an orgasm; it is also theirs.

Many factors are at play; your partner could be stressed and worried about everyday things or needs to communicate more effectively what they like and don't like.

In addition, there are various situations in which not having an orgasm is part of the sexual practice. For example, some men get excited by having their orgasms controlled by their partners and being continually denied the chance to have one.

In short, not being able to make your partner have an orgasm is not drama; you can do better the next time or continue playing. In a sexual relationship, more than one person is involved, and pleasure and responsibility are divided equally.

These are just some of the more common negative sex beliefs I have encountered throughout my career that can prevent us from connecting with our dark feminine energy. Unfortunately, covering them all with a single book is obviously impossible, and sometimes the intervention of a sexuality counselor is recommended to have a personalized recovery path.

Now, let's leave negative sexual beliefs behind us, and in the next chapter, let's focus on the dark feminine seduction.

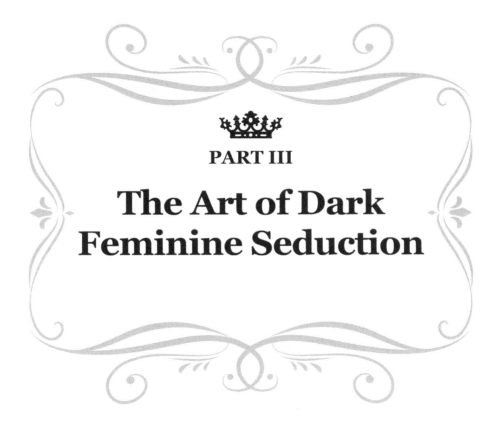

PART III

The Art of Dark Feminine Seduction

ow that you learned various ways to connect with your dark feminine energy, it is time to put these newly acquired skills into action. This part will be about how to put the art of seduction at your service. How does seduction work? How do men work? What are the steps to make someone obsessed with you?

Once you have acquired knowledge about men and how to seduce them, it will be up to you how to use these skills.

Some dear friends wanted to learn more about seduction to win their exes back. Others wanted to use the dark feminine energy as a weapon for revenge, flirting with men for pleasure and leaving them unsatisfied and miserable when the right time came! I do not recommend approaching the dark feminine energy to win your ex back. It is not worth the effort and energy to win back someone that didn't appreciate what he had in the first place. You shouldn't even consider being with someone who doesn't see your value!

One thing I learned while channeling my inner femme fatale is that if someone doesn't see my value, they don't deserve me.

So, I understand women who want to use their dark feminine energy for these purposes. But allow me to warn you, that path leads mostly to unhappiness. The need for revenge or to win someone's love back are manifestations of wounded energy. Of course, you want to cause trouble because you are hurt, but this approach will only make you feel worse about yourself. So, instead of revenge, you should focus on healing your wounds, resetting your energy, and moving on. You may think that only your ex-partner can help you to heal. I used to believe that, but that is a big lie. Once something is broken, it can never return as it was. So, do not let the past affect your future and your happiness. If you are hurt, you should focus on healing; love can do that, and I am not talking about the love that comes from others. I am talking about the love you should feel for yourself! It's precisely what a femme fatale does! She loves herself, and she puts herself first! She doesn't allow disrespectful men to play with her. She is the one who plays with them because she knows how men's psychology works, and more importantly, she knows her actual value!

It doesn't mean the femme fatale doesn't put herself in long relationships. If she cares about someone who appreciates and treats her respectfully, they can end up together for a long time. A woman who reaches her full potential can decide to do whatever she wants in the relationships with the men she seduces. If you are looking for short and fun adventures, want to find the man of your life, or wish to spice up your current relationship, dark feminine energy can help in any decisions you make. Remember, you are doing this for yourself, not for others. You are learning to reach the better version of yourself!

CHAPTER 8

A Brief Journey Into the Male Psyche

Women have discovered that they cannot rely on men's
chivalry to give them justice.
–Helen Keller

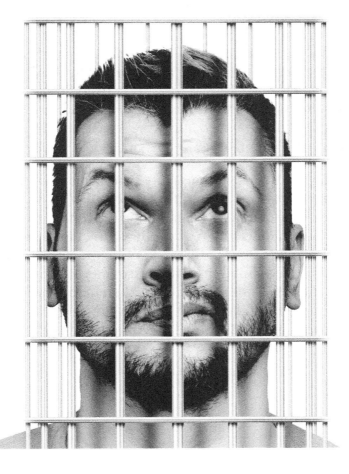

To be able to affect others with your dark feminine energy, you need to understand men's thinking processes. Let's start by saying there are some misconceptions about women's and men's psyches.

We are used to hearing that boys and girls are from two different planets. *Men are from Mars, Women are from Venus*, like the title of John Gray's bestseller, first published in the early 1990s. But recent studies revealed that it is often a mistake to assume that gender differences are rooted in the brain. While physical differences are evident between genders, we cannot take a person's psyche for granted by knowing only their gender. People's behaviors and thoughts depend on their upbringing, education, and traumas.

If you have a specific target in your mind that you want to seduce, knowing his past and childhood is a significant help to understanding his personality and behaviors. So, if your target is someone you have known for a long time, it will be easy for you to understand his psyche and plan your actions to get closer to him. But digging into someone's past may be creepy and inappropriate for someone we have just met.

Fortunately for us, we already know our society's expectations, so we know how men were raised when they were children. If women are to be obedient, elegant, and quiet, men must be sturdy, reliable, and efficient. We tell the young boys not to cry and act tough, while the girls are to be polite and graceful. All these constraints have shaped their mind from a young age, influencing their thoughts and behavior in their adult lives. All these expectations generate patterns in men's minds that we can use for our purposes, and I will tell you about them in this chapter.

MEN WANT TO FEEL USEFUL

Speaking of men's psyche, the need to feel useful and responsible is one characteristic that emerges first in men. Since society has accustomed them to be the breadwinners who will care for the rest of the family, it is crucial for a man to feel useful. Even though culture has changed, giving women more space, a man's need to feel helpful is essential to his ego; this explains why men hesitate to call the plumber or the handyman when there is some chore to do at home.

This behavior is what psychologist James Baurer calls "hero instinct" in his book *His Secret Obsession*. The author attributes this name because the sensation perceived by the man being useful is comparable to the hero who saves the damsel in distress. They like the feeling of saving the day! When a man does not feel needed in a relationship, it is difficult for him to build a strong connection with his partner.

Fortunately for us, this behavior is in sync with our dark feminine energy. The femme fatale in us likes to be treated like a queen! She is independent but also wants to feel appreciated and is inclined to accept any kind gesture from a guy. Again, feminine energy is about receiving, while masculine energy is giving. So, let him lend you his jacket if you feel cold, or let him pay for dinner. If he does not take the initiative, you can send signals by saying, "it is pretty cold here," while looking him in the eyes, or saying, "my bag is quite heavy!" so they can propose to carry it (they usually like to feel strong and masculine!) The chapter in this book dedicated to body language will come in handy for this type of communication. However, my final suggestion is to avoid being explicit in your requests. As a femme fatale, you want to keep the veil of mystery and appear independent. Directly asking for something would ruin the appeal of your dark energy. Therefore, throw implicit messages, and let him come to you as a gentleman. If he does not understand, he probably does not have enough attraction for you, or maybe he is just not particularly receptive!

MEN ARE MORE SENSITIVE THAN WOMEN

I know! This may sound unrealistic and unbelievable, but some researchers prove it true! For example, in 2014, a marketing company named Mindlab applied a test to measure the difference in emotional reactions between the two genders. The experiment involved the same number of women and men who were monitored while watching some videos, in which content was categorized into four different topics. The results showed that men felt stronger emotions than women; the same conclusion appeared in all four categories.

What is even more interesting, however, is comparing these data with the answers men gave when they were asked to express their emotions just after the vision of those videos. Based on their reply, men's feelings seemed less intense than women's, but the result from the electrodes on their skin proved the opposite.

From this test, we can assume that men tend to suppress their feelings, but they are as sensitive as women, and probably even more. Neuropsychologist Dr. David Lewis, the director of Mindlab, said: "This study suggests that men feel emotion just as much as women, sometimes more strongly, but are less willing to express these emotions openly due to expectations put on them by society."

This knowledge can be potent in attracting a man emotionally. Imagine being in their shoes, spending your whole life suppressing feelings because society wants you to act tough. If I had to do that, I would not manage the pressure, honestly. I would be grumpy most of the time! In these circumstances, girls are probably luckier than boys because, at least, they can express themselves freely and let all their emotions come out.

But men are also human beings, so they sometimes must let these feelings out. The best thing we can do to help is to give them space. The worst thing is to pressure them to open! Men must feel safe before opening up; forcing them will only make them uncomfortable! Be patient if you want to win their confidence, especially if you have just met. It will require time before a man can feel genuinely safe around you.

Another suggestion I'd like to share is not to blame your man when he makes stupid mistakes. Reconnecting to the fact that men are sensitive, they can also be very touchy. They can get offended quickly if their pride and dignity are under threat, with the result that they may eventually run away. If you want to keep your target's attention, do not shout at him, and never disrespect him in front of others. Instead, try to be supportive. You can tell him he did something wrong but also that mistakes can happen and that it's not the end of the world! Sometimes, if the atmosphere gets too intense and you think he realizes what he did wrong, you can try to make a laugh out of it. A woman with a sense of humor is always more attractive than one who constantly screams and complains. You'll be surprised at the results you can achieve without taking a situation head-on! This tip obviously applies to innocent mistakes due to carelessness or good faith, like forgetting his wallet or even the anniversary! Mistakes like cheating or being disrespectful are not even contemplated. If this is your case, I urge you to walk away from him ASAP. A dark feminine doesn't waste her time with people who are not worth it.

You may wonder, "What about if I get angry, and I do not want to laugh off the little mistakes he has made?" It depends on how your feelings may affect your behavior. If you feel like making a scene, walk away and give yourself time to calm down. If you can keep yourself together and act normally, express your feelings to your partner privately. This is what a femme fatale would do!

MEN ARE HOPELESS ROMANTICS

Recent surveys prove that men in North America tend to fall in love before women do; they are also the first to say "I love you" at the beginning of a relationship.

A survey published in the Journal of Social Psychology by Marissa A. Harrison and Jennifer C. Shortal interviewed 172 students between boys and girls. Despite the expectation of 9 out of 10 people with experience in previous relationships that it's likely for women to fall in love first, the final data showed that men are the first to fall in love and that three times as many men as women said, "I love you" first to their partners.

Sure, the survey was conducted only between students, but a more recent study conducted in 2022 involved 1400 participants of different ages and from around the world. The conclusion was that men usually say "I love you" before women do (Watkins, 2022). The same study showed that men are the first to say the three words even when the study population contains mostly women. In other words, men express their love first to their partner despite having more choices, probably because they genuinely mean it.

If you wonder how long it takes for both genders to say the "L" word, the same research revealed that the average time for men is around 97.3 days, while it's about 138 days for women. Also, men consider a confession of love acceptable after one month into dating, while women prefer to wait until two or three months.

It is important to note that, statistically, men tend to respond negatively if the partner confesses her love after sex. Instead, they are more likely to respond positively if the confession comes before sex because they see the relationship moving toward physical intimacy. The opposite is for women. The female gender is skeptical when the "I love you" words come before sex because it seems like a way to rush into bed. However, they tend to respond positively if the confession comes after sex because it could signal an interest in a long commitment.

Now that you know that men are hopeless romantics, you can use this information to your advantage. For example, if you are looking just for physical intimacy and not for a long commitment, you now know that men tend to fall in love just after a month from when you start dating. Therefore, I suggest being honest with him from the beginning of the relationship, sharing your boundaries, and ensuring he understands them. If you want to avoid long commitments, tell him directly on the first or second date and ensure you are both on the same page! When you date him, keep the encounters on a physical level and don't get emotionally involved; otherwise, he may think you've reconsidered your decision, and he may search for something more.

If, on the other hand, you want to face a long relationship with your partner, you are now aware that men appreciate women who express their feelings before having sex. However, I suggest you don't rush.

A dark feminine knows what she wants and how to get it. Expressing everything you feel too soon could put you in a position of weakness where partners interested only in manipulating you could take advantage.

Instead, you can keep your man hooked and play with him until you feel ready to say the magic words. You must introduce yourself a little at a time to keep him interested. Don't get lost in long speeches; always keep a veil of mystery. Instead of rushing into a love confession, let him know that you enjoy spending time with him, express that you feel safe around him, and appreciate all the little attentions he gives you. Remember that men love to feel gratified. Lastly, when complimenting your partner, avoid being trivial and make it personal. For example, if you're dating a gym guy, he's probably used to getting praise for his body. But if you notice something unique about him that few people know, your compliment will have a greater impact. For example, if you realize he's a dog lover, you can tell him: "I love that little smirk you get every time you see a dog." These small details will keep his interest alive and let him know that you are serious about your intentions with him.

CHAPTER 9

How to Make Men Obsess Over You

Justice is about making sure that being polite is not the same
thing as being quiet. In fact, oftentimes, the most righteous
thing you can do is shake the table.
—Alexandria Ocasio-Cortez

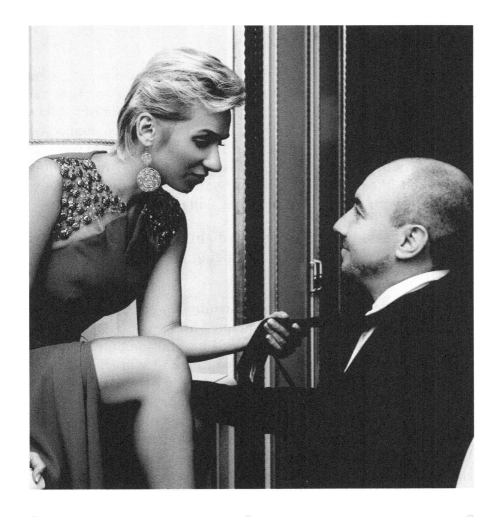

ow that you've learned how to manage your dark feminine energy and have a basic knowledge of the man's psyche, it's time to try your skills in the field. In this section, I will give you tips for getting noticed by the man you want to attract and how to keep his interest alive. If you are already dating a person of your interest, you can skip the first section of this chapter as I reveal some tricks to get you noticed. From the subsection *"Master the Allure of Mystery"*, I will instead provide you with some tricks to keep him hooked and make you the only person he dreams of.

A Dark Feminine Never Woos But Allows Herself To Be Wooed.

You don't want the man you like to think you're desperate to be noticed; instead, you want him to come to you! Taking the first step to getting to know someone is a characteristic of masculine energy. To channel your feminine energy, let the men come to you. This will put you in a position of power where you can decide whether to accept the courtship. It doesn't matter how much you like a person; don't put yourself at a disadvantage; wait, play your cards right, and they will come to you.

If you break this rule, you will have already lost a part of your charm, and it will be more challenging to get his interest and make him obsess over you!

You have to create the right opportunity to get noticed by the man you like. For this reason, you must find a way to get into one of his circles first. Try to understand his routine and interests. If he's a coworker, time your coffee or cigarette break to match his. If he frequents a specific pub, try going there more often with your friends, or subscribe to his gym or a class where he is registered too. You have to shorten the distance but never address him directly. He must not suspect that you are around for him. Your presence should feel casual and spontaneous. Essentially, you're giving him the possibility to make the first move.

If you want to get near him in a public place, I suggest you go with a friend or a group of friends. That way, he won't suspect you're there for him. Surrounding yourself with people you already know will not only help you keep your cover intact but also help with your confidence.

GET NOTICED BY HIM

Once you get into one of his circles, it is time to use your charm to get noticed by him. Here are some suggestions that will help get his attention:

- **Don't hide behind the corner.** You have to let your potential man notice you! So, don't isolate yourself by looking at your cell phone the whole time or standing still doing nothing. Refrain from giving the impression that you wish to be somewhere else. Instead, try to be active within his circle. Ask questions showing interest if you're at a class or business meeting. If you're at a party, be involved in conversations. I'm not saying you have to put yourself on stage; far from it. A femme fatale avoids the spotlight yet knows how to get noticed. You don't want to appear bored when he is in his environment if you want to be seen by him. Look interested and slightly excited to be there; he will notice you.

- **Get your friends involved.** Remember when I said to go to a place he frequents with one or more friends? This is not only a perfect way to avoid making it clear to everyone that you are there for him, but it will also help to put yourself in a brighter light. Being surrounded by people who respect and esteem you will help you bring out the best side of yourself and appear more attractive in the eyes of those who see you from the outside. Having fun with your friends will be one of your strategies to get his attention. And if this or other tactics don't work, you can always trust one of your companions to introduce you to the person you're targeting. In this way, you will have acquired your target without approaching him directly.

- **Talk to everyone but him.** Pretend you didn't even notice him. Talk to everyone in the room but don't go to him. If you've done your homework correctly and made him interested in you, he'll wonder why you are ignoring him. These thoughts will make him curious and nervous. Men are very competitive and seeing you talking to everyone and avoiding him will increase his desire and obsession to know you. At this point, if he's not shy and has an interest in you, he'll come forward to get your attention.

- **Use your body language to show confidence and poise.** Power posing and how you use your hands and eyes are all important factors to stand out in the crowd. The chapter on body language will surely help you in this regard.

- **Make him believe that he is hitting on you.** The points listed above must lead to this conclusion. Make your man believe that hitting on you was his idea! You may have realized how competitive a man can be, and this will be the secret to your success! To make a man obsess over you, you must convince him that your relationship started because of him. He was the one who noticed you and approached you first. He was the one who won your attention and feelings among dozens of competitors. He is the chosen one who now has the privilege to spend time with you. Of course, you will know that you juggled everything to make it happen but allow him to believe that he conquered you. Men love challenges and dating a woman who is already flirting with them will be a too-easy game. Instead, they want the competition. They want to feel like they are unique and superior to other men. A femme fatale knows this little trick and how to use it to get the men she wants.

Master the Allure of Mystery

The mystery around a dark feminine is essential for her magnetism. The less we know about a person, the more we are intrigued by them, especially if that individual is attractive, confident, and successful.

Obviously, the mystery alone is not enough. A person we don't know much who is shy, insecure, and humble doesn't leave a strong first impression. The allure of mystery works well in synergy with perceived confidence. The more you are confident, the more people will be intrigued by how much they don't know about you.

For this reason, I recommend combining the exercises in part two with the advice in this section if you want to grow your dark feminine skills altogether.

Now, how can you be mysterious with the person you're dating? The short answer is to reveal yourself gradually; the execution is more complex.

Many women make the mistake of oversharing from the beginning of their relationship. For example, they reveal everything about their life on the first date or send long messages getting anxious if the receiver doesn't reply within 10 minutes. You may think that being constantly in touch with your lover helps to keep his interest alive, but it is more likely to lead to the opposite effect. Also, this will put you in a weak position where he will feel like you desperately need him. Instead, if you want your date to remain infatuated with you, you have to learn to carefully guard who you are and share just enough to keep him on the hook. Following are some tips for building and maintaining an aura of mystery.

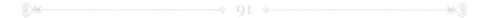

Keep Conversations Short

When a man wants to get to know you, you don't have to tell everything about yourself on the first date. I understand that the thrill of dating the man you had targeted can rush you to talk about your whole life, but you must resist the temptation and be more inclined to listen than to speak. Be a good listener and a short talker; curiosity is a strong emotion, and giving up such a powerful weapon would be a waste.

For this reason, try to say very little about yourself and reveal only enough to keep your listener in suspense until the next date. If you think about it, even directors adopt a similar strategy in some TV series. Have you ever seen an episode that ends with a cliffhanger? Just when you were caught up in the climax and couldn't wait to watch what would come next. It leaves you a little disappointed for a bit, but how intense is the curiosity to see the following episode? If you're lucky enough to have the entire series at your disposal, you've probably already started the next episode (and this is how I ended my favorite series on Netflix in only three days!) But if the show releases one episode a week, you'll spend the next seven days thinking about it, getting increasingly impatient as the days go by.

As TV directors, even the dark feminine is a good storyteller. To keep your audience hooked, you don't have to tell the whole story at once. Instead, divide it into the most intriguing episodes and reveal them precisely at the right time. Doing so will increase your magnetism and make your date eager to see you again.

I understand that this approach is not simple. There is a risk of being boring if you limit yourself to a few words. Don't worry; the following tips are going to help you!

- **Prepare your topics.** To avoid being boring, prepare for the various topics that the discussion could fall on and what you want to share with your listener. For example, decide in advance to share your holiday in Greece if the opportunity arises, but save your road trip in Australia for the next occasion. This preparatory work will also allow you to decide how to structure the conversation around the various topics to sell yourself in the best possible way.

- **Let them prompt for more details.** You don't have to go into detail when someone asks you a personal question. But of course, you can't ignore the question completely; for example, if someone asks you about your hobbies, you can answer, "I like water sports," without having to specify that you have been going to the pool regularly three times a week since you were six years old. If it is not part of your preparation work, play it safe. If the guy is interested, he will ask you more questions. Remember that communication is not limited to spoken words alone; the messages you send him must also respect this rule. It would make little sense to prepare your conversations during dates accurately, and then send him long texts when you do not see each other. Doing so would make you look more eager than mysterious. Use texting wisely, share only what you feel is needed, and do your best to sell it well.

- **Make your body language prevail over speech.** The power of speech is often overrated. A look or a gesture can be more than enough to express yourself. Applying body language instead of speaking is preferable when you want to minimize your communication. That's why I devoted an entire section to non-verbal communication.

- **Learn to be a better listener.** A quality of the dark feminine is the ability to leave room for others. You should not try to steal the spotlight; you should let the spotlight come to you at the right time. Listening is a learning opportunity; it allows you to study the situation and find the perfect timing and way to join the discussion. Also, others will see you interested in what they say and treat you more favorably. So, from now on, try to listen more and speak a bit less.

Time Is Your Best Ally

A femme fatale knows that time is a scarce resource, so she hardly gives hers to others if it's not worth it. It might go unnoticed by the inattentive observer, but time plays a fundamental role in the seduction game.

For instance, think about what I said before about revealing yourself little by little; it is still a matter of time. You don't tell everything about yourself immediately, but you do it on a mental schedule. The dark feminine is patient and uses time in her favor, and you can master it too.

Here are some tricks that will help you.

- **Show a busy schedule.** Everyone should be aware of how highly you regard your time. As a woman always looking to improve herself, you live a busy life filled with passions and interests. Take your time when you need to confirm a date, even if you know you are available. Don't respond "yes" to the guy you like when he asks you out because that suggests you weren't waiting for anything else. Be calm and answer that you need to double-check your schedule and will confirm later. People should understand that you will only spend time with those who deserve your presence but also that you have no problem moving on without them.

- **Take your time.** People can be very impatient, particularly in the early stage of a relationship. One of the most common mistakes is constantly checking your phone and responding as soon as a message arrives. This compulsive behavior shows that you have nothing better to do than check your phone, making you appear desperate and insecure. Instead, your goal is establishing yourself as a busy and confident but still approachable woman, so you should learn to take your time. Reply to messages only after a few hours. Cut long texting conversations if they are leading to nowhere. Someone who wants to see or hear from you must accept that you also have other commitments, and your life doesn't revolve around them. You can show some flexibility, but you come first. If you think making someone wait is impolite, it's because you tend to use light energy. We've already established that a dark female prioritizes herself first, so she doesn't mind taking the time and space she needs. Consider that waiting is not always bad for a man; instead, it is a way to test his tenacity and confirm his genuine interest in a woman. Remember that some men enjoy a challenge, while those who are not really interested will change targets at the first obstacle. For those who enjoy a small challenge, waiting will make them even more impatient to hear from you.

- **Be patient.** You can only use time to your advantage if you're patient. A femme fatale is a strategist. We see her getting everything she wants with little effort in the movies, but life is not a movie. Patience is a virtue that the dark feminine uses on various occasions. If you want a solid and long lasting relationship, patience is key. Give your partner the same space that you would like for yourself. Don't get upset if he doesn't respond to your messages immediately. Like you, he has his interests and his needs. Let him know if he crosses one of your boundaries, but do not ever overreact. Most exercises this book suggests will also help you improve your patience. Self-reflection and self-compassion exercises are especially beneficial. Being more self-aware also means being more tolerant of others. A dark feminine is always composed and in control, no matter what.

Be Unpredictable

Being unpredictable is another crucial aspect of being mysterious. You don't want to be a dull woman with a set routine. Those who are repetitive run the risk of becoming boring. We've already stated that men enjoy a good challenge, and you should always keep your men on their toes!

When I say you have to be unpredictable, I don't mean you can't plan your life and give up any routine. I'm just suggesting that you don't get entirely tied to your agenda and goals and leave room for something unexpected. Adding some randomness to your life will make you more attractive to those who know you and keep your life more interesting.

Here are some tips to make yourself unpredictable.

- **Have a flexible routine.** A routine is an excellent way to develop good habits, but you can embed some flexibility into it. For example, if a friend invites you to breakfast and you really want to go, but you usually exercise at the gym in the morning, you can reschedule your workout for later. Taking the liberty to change your routine and adjust it to your needs demonstrates security and adaptability. You affirm that you are a woman who does not live in a box but allows herself some freedom to fulfill both her pleasures and her duties. Missing some appointments is also a way to show love to the people in your life. People who know how busy you are and how much you care about fulfilling your commitments will understand how much you value them when you adapt your agenda to fit them in your life. However, make it happen only on rare occasions, or it won't be a routine anymore. If you cancel an appointment for someone, it's because, for once, you prefer their company to your obligations. You do deserve some fun once in a while! Use this little gesture of affection with the people you care about the most, but avoid doing it with people you've recently met, particularly boyfriends you've been dating for a few weeks. If you skip your commitments to date a new boyfriend, he will believe he has you at his complete disposal, putting him in a dominant position.

- **Be open-minded.** An open-minded person is willing to consider new cultures and opportunities. It will be easier for you to get involved and find alternative activities if you are open to new points of view and new adventures. Open-minded people are willing to step outside their comfort zone to face new challenges and learn from new experiences. Someone open to novelty is an unpredictable person who can come up with brilliant ideas and contemplations that a person stuck in their comfort zone could not consider. To embrace your dark feminine energy, you must strive to be open-minded. This way, you can discover new interests and improve your current self. Leaving the comfort zone is always a risk and an effort. An easy way to get out of it without stress is to rediscover the activities you enjoyed as a child. Your brain will associate these activities with memories; they will feel familiar enough to make you feel at ease. Rediscovering what you enjoyed doing when you were younger can reawaken interests that you had forgotten about and may want to pursue again. Another way to step out of the box is to do something completely unexpected, even by your standards. In my case, I was watching The Greatest Showman for the 100th time when, thanks to a scene in the movie, I decided on the destination of my next holiday. Do you remember when the protagonist rides an elephant to the train station to meet the rest of the family? At that moment, I decided I wanted to try elephant riding too. Two months later, we were in India.

- **Make your dates challenging.** Invite your lover to unusual appointments to make yourself even more mysterious and intriguing in his eyes. The femme fatale is a resourceful woman who always surprises you. Therefore, you want your time with him to be varied and exciting. Sure, having a romantic dinner is nice, but occasionally try unusual and intriguing ideas. Several studies have found that people easily remember the unusual and often have intense feelings associated with it. Endorphins like adrenaline stimulate the senses, making recalling facts and people from those events easier. If you want your man to have vivid memories of you, to the point of obsession, plan breathtaking activities with him. Something exciting but also a little frightening. You may think I would suggest some risky activities, like skydiving and bungee jumping. These options undoubtedly provide intense emotions, but it's understandable if you don't want to risk your life for a bit of fun. Without jumping into extreme sports, other activities release endorphins, such as dancing, hiking, and scuba diving. If you are not inclined to sports, you will be pleased to know that spicy food also releases endorphins. Therefore, a meal at an Indian or Mexican restaurant can be a valid option.

Allow His Inner Self to Come Out!

In psychology and sociology, the mask is a recurring theme. It is the most appropriate metaphor to explain how an individual changes personality based on the context as if wearing a mask. Of course, the contexts are different: family, work, friends, the supermarket, the golf club, and so on. Every social context has its rules, and we must adjust our behavior, thoughts, and sometimes values to be accepted.

> *A person tends to wear a mask when he is in the presence of others and to lay it aside when he is alone. The mask used in society is that of standardized expressive equipment. It is a typical defense used by the individual against the possible threat of embarrassment or failure. The mask is that which arrests the eye, and the body beneath it is irrelevant* (Erving Goffman, The Presentation of Self in Everyday Life, 1959).

But behind the mask is a repressed inner child. I'm not talking specifically about your man. Still, I'm referring to a branch of psychology that, oversimplifying, addresses the subconscious as the "inner child," which is the individual's most authentic and genuine part. The inner child is someone's true identity suppressed over time to assert himself in society and is also the most vulnerable part of our being.

It is difficult for men to express their emotions with others because it is an attitude that is hardly tolerated by the society in which we live. Therefore, men must feel protected and safe to open up. They must be sure not to be "attacked" when they are most vulnerable.

To truly conquer a man, you should make him feel comfortable expressing himself. He has to trust that he can drop any masks and reveal his true personality when alone with you. Give your man time to open up and show him that he can trust you. Don't judge him when he is vulnerable; support him on these occasions. If he sees that you are honest with him, he will be more encouraged to show himself. As you can understand, it's not an easy and immediate process, but if you manage to be part of his comfort zone, you will have conquered the keys to his heart!

CHAPTER 10

Develop a Magnetic Body Language

Fearlessness is like a muscle. I know from my own life that the more I exercise it, the more natural it becomes to not let my fears run me.
—Arianna Huffington

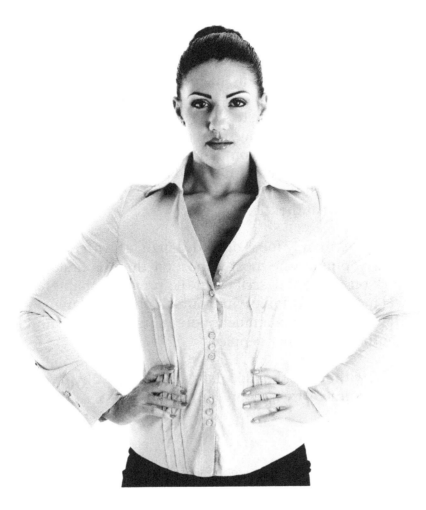

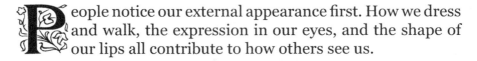

People notice our external appearance first. How we dress and walk, the expression in our eyes, and the shape of our lips all contribute to how others see us.

Have you ever found yourself judging a person by their physical appearance? How do they walk? How comfortable or uncomfortable do they seem when doing a certain action?

Judging someone based on their appearance is common, and we often do it without even realizing it. This chapter will focus on the perception that others have of you to help you externalize your transformation into a femme fatale.

The main objective of this section is to help you interact easily with other people, be able to convey your boundaries, and arouse a magnetic attraction in your possible partners.

Using your body language to show the world your inner femme fatale can be a powerful way to access your dark feminine energy while expressing your confidence and sexiness. But remember not to overdo it. One of the fundamental characteristics of those in tune with their dark female energy is to feel comfortable and appear authentic.

Some coaches mainly focus on body language with their clients, but in my opinion, the most important thing is first to do all the work on yourself described in the previous chapters. Once you feel more comfortable with yourself, the body language of a dark feminine will come much more naturally to you and look more authentic to other people.

And now, without further ado, let's start talking about the manners that characterize a femme fatale.

POWER POSES

The first thing I want to discuss is **power poses**. A power pose is a technique that quickly boosts your confidence and changes your state of mind.

According to a study published in the Psychological Science Journal (Carney, 2010):

> *Posing in high-power non-verbal displays (as opposed to low-power non-verbal displays) would cause neuroendocrine and behavioral changes for both male and female: [...]posing in displays of power causes advantaged and adaptive psychological and behavioral changes, and these findings suggest that embodiment extends beyond mere thinking and feeling, to physiology and subsequent behavioral choices. That a person can, by assuming two simple 1-min poses, embody power and instantly become more powerful has real-world, actionable implications.*

Power posing is based on taking up space and asserting dominance with your presence. In our primitive brain, a person who takes up space with confidence automatically seems more important than one who curls up in a corner.

You can use various power poses to seem more confident:

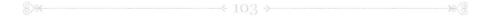

1. Stand upright with your hands resting on your hips to convey a feeling of security and dominance.

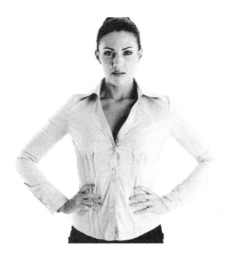

2. If you are in a meeting room or near a table or desk and the situation is suitable, you can use this power pose to assert dominance. Stand up with the table before you and elegantly place your hands on it, touching it only with your fingertips. Then, lean forward slightly as if to approach people around the table.

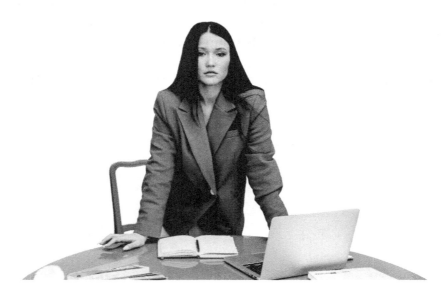

3. Based on the situation, try to adopt a posture that takes up more space when you sit down. Obviously, in a formal dinner, there is a certain etiquette to follow, but in more informal situations, sitting in one of the following postures can convey a sense of dominance and create a strong interest in possible partners.

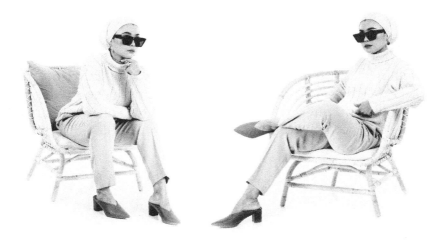

4. The **thinker pose** is frequently used by celebrities like former President Obama and Oprah Winfrey. It consists in holding your fingertips together to convey authority.

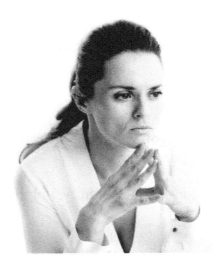

Another aspect to consider concerning body language is the **default posture**. For example, standing tall and straight is essential to appear confident, as if an invisible string connects the top of your head and the ceiling. Also, while adopting this posture, your chin must always be kept up. The challenge is not maintaining this posture but looking relaxed and comfortable.

As already said, anyone can play the part of the femme fatale, but few can genuinely feel like one. Being relaxed and not seeming stiff and awkward takes practice. Working on what is suggested in part two of the book *How to Tap Into Your Dark Feminine Energy* can help you feel more natural when using your dark feminine energy. Without developing self-confidence, it won't be easy to be credible and feel comfortable with this new body language.

IT IS ALL IN YOUR HANDS

Your hands are a powerful medium to convey confidence and charisma. The first rule to remember is:

don't hide your hands!

Your hand positions can communicate a variety of messages. Instead of hiding your hands during a conversation, use them to reinforce the message you want to convey.

Here are some basic poses that might be helpful to you.

1. **Lowered steeple position** shows that you are listening with interest but simultaneously showing confidence. Angela Merkel (former Chancellor of Germany) is famous for often using this hand position.

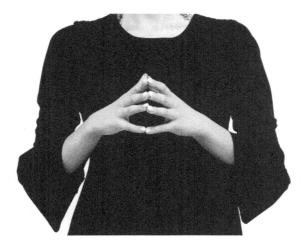

2. **The limp wrist** is handy when showing temporary weakness or a sign of attraction. If used on a date, it can convey to the man the idea that the woman is submissive, and he can assume a more dominant role. I don't recommend using this gesture frequently, but this position could be advantageous when you want the man to take the initiative.

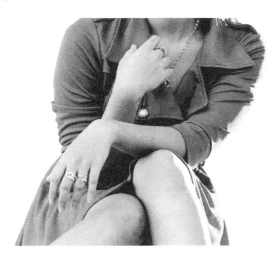

3. **Touch me, please**, is not a hand gesture but a way to transfer the desire to touch someone to an inanimate object. It's a way to show the urge to touch someone without saying it openly. For example, imagine you're on a first date and holding a glass of champagne. You're having a brilliant conversation, you like him, and you want to let him know you're ready to go beyond just talking. One way to demonstrate this is to hold the glass prominently in front of you, and while maintaining the same tone of the conversation, start running your fingers slowly over the glass as if you were touching his body.

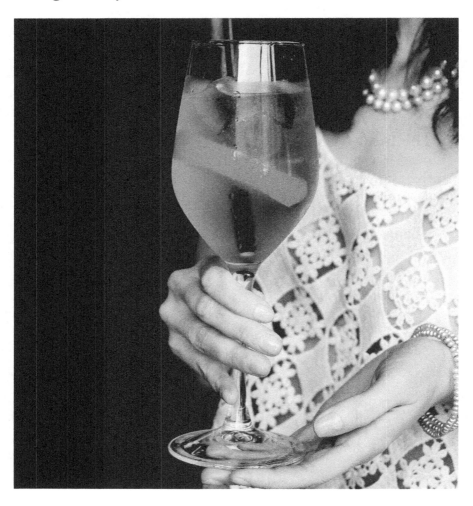

4. **I'm ready.** It is a gesture used during a speech to capture people's attention. It shows that you have something to say and are ready to say it. Your hands are open and well in sight, and your gaze is fixed on your listeners.

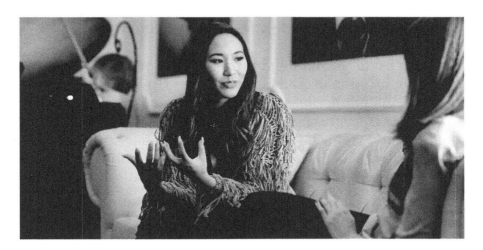

5. **Open palm and exposed wrist:** I decided to include this hand position in the list not because it is part of those adopted by a femme fatale but because I want you to know its meaning to avoid adopting it when you want to convey security. The man's brain can interpret a woman who exposes her palm and wrists as weak and submissive.

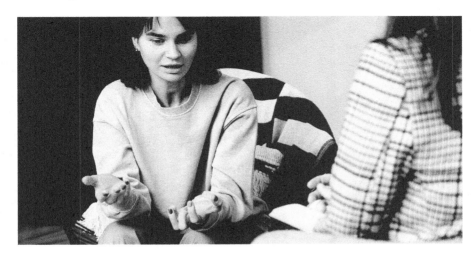

Don't Show Your Weakness

The "open palm and exposed wrist" and "the limp wrist" are not the only elements of a woman's body language that show vulnerability and submission. Other elements should be avoided or used consciously and only in certain situations.

Here is a list of the main indicators that a woman is shy, shows vulnerability, or takes a defensive stance. Obviously, I am illustrating them not because I invite you to adopt them but rather to see if you recognize yourself in some of these attitudes. Next time you find yourself (not intentionally) in one of these poses, try to switch to a power pose, and you may notice a tiny improvement in your confidence.

1. **Crossing arms:** Men and women widely use this position to assume a defensive attitude. Crossing arms is usually adopted when a person is losing an argument, or they are under pressure. If you ever find yourself in these situations, try to adopt a more open and relaxed position instead of crossing your arms. Leave your hands at your sides slightly out from your body to show openness and confidence.

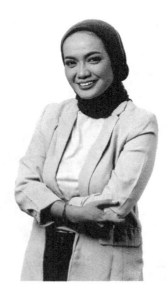

2. **Locked ankles:** Although, according to etiquette, it is good practice for a woman to use this seated posture when wearing a skirt, locking the ankles can also convey nervousness and vulnerability. Try instead to cross your legs; to immediately feel sexier and more self-confident.

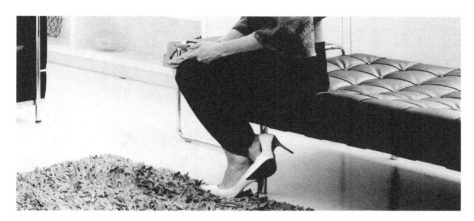

3. **Lip biting:** Although biting the lips in movies is often associated with desire, the reality is very different. You can seduce a man with your lips, but you must be careful how you use your eyes. Sensually biting the lips in combination with intense eye contact is a way of expressing strong desire. On the other hand, biting your lips with little or no eye contact totally changes the message. In this second case, the man may interpret this behavior as stress or anxiety.

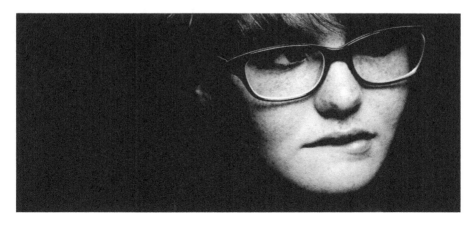

4. **Touching your face or neck:** Repeatedly touching your face or neck during a conversation indicates that you are not in control of the conversation and do not feel comfortable. Try to keep your hands away from your face while interacting with someone.

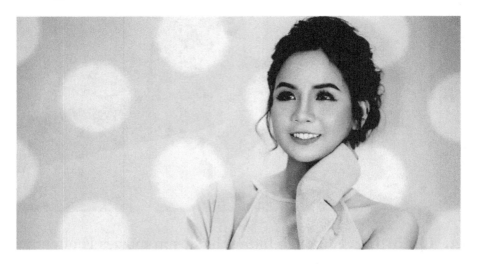

5. **Making yourself small:** If there is one thing to avoid doing, it is to make yourself small. Standing tall with a high chin and straight shoulders is essential to projecting confidence. Also, don't fold your arms or hold your elbow.

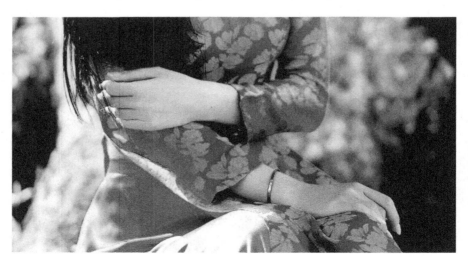

THE POWER OF EYES

The phrase "the eyes are the windows to the soul" can be interpreted as the idea that one can know a person's thoughts and secrets just by looking into their eyes.

Obviously, the reality is quite different, but the eyes play a fundamental role in non-verbal communication and are an integral part of our body language.

Compared to the rest of our body, we have less control over the eyes, the pupils can dilate involuntarily, or the eyelids flutter more rapidly, perhaps indicating a stressful situation in contrast to well-controlled body language. In short, the eyes can be your best allies, enhancing the non-verbal message you want to send or betraying nervousness and insecurities. So, let's see what to do and not to do with the eyes to convey the messages you want.

- **Make extra eye contact:** Establishing eye contact with the person you want to seduce is positive since it shows interest and confidence simultaneously. Insecure women tend not to make enough eye contact with the person they are talking to or always look away first.

- **Look at the mouth:** This is a very effective move because when you want to kiss someone, you tend to look at the mouth of the person. This is a way of evoking the feeling of the kiss in both your mind and your potential partner. He will have the impression that you want to kiss him, even if you are just sitting at a table on a date.

- **Eye rolling:** This is a no-no! Eye-rolling is a symptom of impatience. This gesture indicates that you are putting effort into keeping frustration at bay. Instead of eye-rolling, it is better to look away for a second, calm down, and assume a power pose before continuing the conversation.

- **Dilated eyes:** This is a problematic reaction to control but can help read the non-verbal language of a person you are interacting with. Research has proven that people's eyes dilate when they see something they desire. Starting from this idea, when you propose various options to a person, pay attention to their reaction; the dilation of their pupils could help you identify what they really want.

- **Silence and eye contact are a killer combination:** When you don't speak and have firm eye contact, it's perfect for building sensual tension with your partner. If you are on the first date and want to test if there is any chemistry between you and him, just stare him in the eyes, don't say a word, touch your glass as illustrated in the *touch me, please* hand gesture, and see how he reacts. It's a slightly aggressive approach, but it worked well with my husband!

THE CALL OF THE SIREN

The voice is a weapon, and the dark feminine knows how to use it to seduce, convey a sense of authority, or more in general, get what she wants.

The tone of voice is one of the first things we notice about a person, and according to various studies, it influences how we perceive a person. For instance, if we talk about leadership:

> *Both men and women select male and female leaders with lower voices. These findings suggest that men and women with lower-pitched voices may be more successful in obtaining positions of leadership* (Klofstad, 2012).

Also, as a side note, still regarding the perceived leadership:

> *While gender discrimination is an obvious cause of the under-representation of women as leaders, our results suggest that biological differences between the sexes, and our responses to those differences, could potential-*

*ly be an additional factor to consider. More specifical-
ly, because women, on average, have higher-pitched
voices than men, and because higher-pitched female
voices are judged to be weaker, less competent, and
less trustworthy, the characteristics of this vocal signal
could help explain why women are less likely to hold
leadership roles than men* (Klofstad, 2012).

If we leave leadership aside and focus only on actual seduction, various studies show that men find women with a higher tone of voice more sensual. This is because a higher pitch is associated with submission, while a lower tone pitch, as already mentioned, is associated with a more decisive character.

Ok, but then, what should we do with our voice? Unfortunately, the answer is not simple; we must use both high and low registers cleverly.

Here are some tips to make the most of your voice and seduce the person you're interested in.

- **Record yourself:** Changing the tone of voice, cadence, and how you speak is not an easy feat and takes practice. When you try a vocal exercise, record and listen to yourself to gradually improve.

- **Relax:** A stressed person tries to speak louder than normal and to speak at a speed that gives the listener the feeling that the speaker is eager to finish the sentence and run away. Whatever effect you want to give to your voice, first remember to breathe, relax your oral muscles, and approach the conversation in a calm state of mind.

- **Slow and low:** Imagine you are on a first date sipping your drinks at the table. This is the perfect situation to play with the dynamics of how you speak. Lower your voice slightly and slow down the cadence, as if you want to make those moments last longer. Adopt a seated power pose. The combination of voice and body language will convey a confident and dominant image to whoever is watching you. At this point, you can take the initiative and see how your date reacts.

- **Pause a little:** If you're about to say something important and want to draw attention to yourself, use silence. During a speech, a person may lose focus; a brief pause triggers a primordial panic in the listener. Has it ever happened to you at school, you get distracted and immediately regain attention when the teacher stops talking, and silence falls? Have you ever found yourself with that hint of fear that they asked something of you? The principle is the same: if you're about to say something important, use silence to create that little moment of panic that brings the listeners back to focus on you.

- **Use the diaphragm:** You can achieve low tones of voice while sounding smooth and relaxed. To learn to use the diaphragm, vocal coaches suggest lying on your back with your knees slightly bent. When you've found the position, place your hands on your rib cage and breathe through your nose. As you perform this exercise, you should feel your stomach push against your hand as you inhale, and the pressure disappears as you exhale. It takes several attempts but try speaking when you feel you have breathed from your diaphragm. You will hear a completely different tone of voice. Speaking using the diaphragm, you will be able to obtain a low and warm voice, perfect for whispering in the ear of your loved one.

THE SCENT

The scent can be a powerful tool for conveying sensations. The perfume you wear reflects who you are or want to be. For example, a floral, fruity, or fresh scent is ideal for connecting with your light feminine energy. On the other hand, a more intense perfume with notes of wood, leather, or spices channels your dark feminine energy.

The femme fatale uses perfume to stimulate all senses and make a lasting impression. Therefore, they choose the fragrance that best represents themselves and wear it for any occasion. You'll eventually learn to identify a woman in tune with her dark feminine by her signature perfume.

As a woman wanting to tap into both energies, you can pick the best perfume depending on the occasion. When seducing a man, for example, you may want to tap into your dark feminine energy and choose a strong fragrance. Conversely, a fresh perfume is more appropriate for an interview or meeting your boyfriend's family.

The type of perfume to wear depends on your preferences. When expressing your femme fatale, I advise you to find your signature perfume. Having a single scent that connects you to your dark feminine energy makes you feel more at ease in this role. It also gives you a distinct element that others can easily recognize when you are in the dark feminine mode. You should select your signature fragrance based on your tastes. Still, if you don't know where to start, this list can help:

- "Dark Purple" by Montale
- "Very Sexy" by Carolina Herrera
- "Crystal Noir" by Versace
- "Poison" by Dior
- "Coco Noir" by Chanelle

About light energy because most women are naturally drawn to light energy, they enjoy selecting a fragrance based on the event. Mood often influences our decision about perfume when we want to connect with our light. When I feel tired or sad, I prefer to select a peach or cherry blossom scent because it reminds me of summer and helps energize me. If, on the other hand, I'm already in a good mood, vanilla is the most appropriate fragrance to express my light energy.

Conclusion

Dark feminine energy is an incredible ally that, if used appropriately, can totally change our lives. Everything written in this book, from self-care to body language, is a small part of the process that will lead you to access a part of yourself you didn't even know you had. Of course, it takes time and patience to fully understand how to manifest your inner femme fatale but trust me; it's worth it.

One thing I would like you to remember after reading this book is to focus on yourself and prioritize your desires and needs. We only have one life, which is too short to waste by pleasing others.

When I wrote this book, I thought of all the incredible women I've met throughout my career and their struggles. I wanted to make something that could reach as many women as possible and provide them with the support they need to reach their full potential. I wrote the book that a young me should have read to avoid so much pain and frustration.

Our journey has come to an end, and I am aware that I have ambitious goals with this manuscript. It is difficult to significantly impact a person's life with these few pages. Nonetheless, I hope the information contained herein was interesting and valuable and can positively impact how you go about life.

I wish you an exciting and happy future where all your dreams will come true.

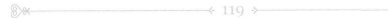

Bonus 1
61 Prompts to Activate Your Dark Feminine Energy

Embark on a transformative journey of self-discovery with our thought-provoking prompts that will awaken your dark feminine energy! Simply scan the QR code or use the URL below to download your bonus.

bit.ly/3IXShPj

Bonus 2
Shadow Work Workbook

Take your journey further with this comprehensive *Shadow Work Workbook*, designed to guide you into discovering your shadow and unleashing your true potential! Simply scan the QR code or use the URL below to download your free Shadow Journal!

bit.ly/3IViQ7D

References

Casey A. Klofstad, Rindy C. Anderson, Susan Peters (2021). Sounds like a winner: voice pitch influences the perception of leadership capacity in both men and women. Proceeding of the Royal Society B: Biological Sciences, 2698-2704

Christopher D. Watkins, J. B. (2022). Men say "I love you" before women do: Robust across several countries.
Journal of Social and Personal Relationships , 2134-2153.

D., D. J. (2017). *Overcoming Religious Sexual Shame.*
Retrieved from Psychology Today: https://www.psychologytoday.com/us/blog/women-who-stray/201708/overcoming-religious-sexual-shame

How to say no. (n.d.). Retrieved from Science of People:
https://www.scienceofpeople.com/how-to-say-no/

How to set boundaries. (n.d.). Retrieved from Science of People:
https://www.scienceofpeople.com/how-to-set-boundaries/

Jacquelyn Crane, F. G. (2010). Optimal Nonverbal Communications Strategies Physicians Should Engage in to Promote Positive Clinical Outcomes. *Health Marketing Quarterly,* 262-274.

Kaufman S. B., J. E. (2020). Healthy Selfishness and Pathological Altruism: Measuring Two Paradoxical Forms of Selfishness.
Frontiers in psychology.

Kent C. Berridge, M. L. (2015). Pleasure systems in the brain.
Neuron, 646-664.

Lee Rowland, O. S. (2018). A range of kindness activities boost happiness.
The Journal of Social Psychology, 340-343.

Lily FitzGibbon, J. K. (2020). The seductive lure of curiosity: information as a motivationally salient reward.
Current Opinion in Behavioral Sciences, 21-27.

Lisa Dawn Hamilton PhD, C. M. (2013). Chronic stress and sexual function in women. *HHS Author Manuscripts*.

Marissa A Harrison, J. C. (2011). Women and Men in Love: Who Really Feels It and Says It First? *The Journal of Social Psychology*, 727-736.

Michela Luciani, M. d. (2022). Measuring self-care in the general adult population: development and psychometric testing of the Self-Care Inventory. *BMC Public Health*.

MK., S. (2019). Masculinity, femininity, and leadership: Taking a closer look at the alpha female. PLoS One.

Sexual_repression. (n.d.). Retrieved from Wikipedia: https://en.wikipedia.org/wiki/Sexual_repression

William J. Chopik, E. S. (2020). Changes in optimism and pessimism in response to life events: Evidence from three large panel studies. *HHS Author Manuscripts*.

Gray, John. *Men are from Mars, Women are from Venus: The Definitive Guide to Relationships*. Element, 2002.

Image References

Alliance Images. (n.d.). At the end of the day, it's all about successfully implementing the strategy and staying true to your vision. Shutterstock. https://www.shutterstock.com/image-photo/end-day-all-about-successfully-implementing-289375949

Andrea Piacquadio. (2020, March 14). Women sitting on couch. Pexels. https://www.pexels.com/photo/women-sitting-on-couch-3937272/

Ariadna22822. (n.d.). Portrait of mysterious beautiful young woman with wonderful skin texture in black hat. Shutterstock. https://www.shutterstock.com/image-photo/portrait-mysterious-beautiful-young-woman-wonderful-176994263

Damon Carter. (n.d.). Angry business woman posing on white background. Shutterstock. https://www.shutterstock.com/image-photo/angry-business-woman-posing-on-white-217776175

Dmitry Lobanov. (n.d.). Brunette woman vamp in off-shoulder dress and with her eyes covered with scarf, blindfold. Shutterstock. https://www.shutterstock.com/image-photo/portrait-brunette-woman-vamp-offshoulder-dress-1949036920

Dominika Roseclay. (2023, February 23). Woman in black one shoulder top holding red carnation. Pexels. https://www.pexels.com/photo/woman-in-black-one-shoulder-top-holding-red-carnation-894754/

FETISH DELUXE. (n.d.). Girl vamp in a mask in a black suit created with feathers. Shutterstock. https://www.shutterstock.com/image-photo/girl-vamp-mask-black-suit-created-229956436

imustbedead. (2011, December 20). Close up of a woman with freckles biting her lip. Pexels. https://www.pexels.com/photo/close-up-of-a-woman-with-freckles-biting-her-lip-10846320/

Marko Aliaksandr. (n.d.). Head of a businessman in a cage. Shutterstock. https://www.shutterstock.com/image-photo/head-businessman-cage-opportunities-limited-business-2148389597

Nadim Sh. (n.d.). A woman holding a cocktail drink. Pexels. https://www.pexels.com/photo/a-woman-holding-a-cocktail-drink-12464906/

PanicAttack. (n.d.). Formal woman in black dress looking at camera with touching fingertips steeple gesture. Shutterstock. https://www.shutterstock.com/image-photo/formal-woman-black-dress-looking-camera-682375924

Prostock-studio. (n.d.). Great appearance, love yourself and perfect skin. Shutterstock. https://www.shutterstock.com/image-photo/great-appearance-love-yourself-perfect-skin-1911438694

RODNAE Productions. (2021, June 29). Woman in blue shirt sitting on black couch. Pexels. https://www.pexels.com/photo/woman-in-blue-shirt-sitting-on-black-couch-9064328/

Ronny Overhate. (n.d.). Woman young beautiful. Pixabay. https://pixabay.com/photos/woman-young-beautiful-pretty-3042408/

RossHelen. (n.d.). Young woman relaxing in the beautiful vintage bath full of foam in the retro bathroom decorated with candles. Shutterstock. https://www.shutterstock.com/image-photo/young-woman-relaxing-beautiful-vintage-bath-776461294

Sewupari Studio. (n.d.). Woman professional portrait smile. Pixabay. https://pixabay.com/photos/woman-professional-portrait-smile-7084055/

shaxlinegraphy. (n.d.). A beautiful Malay girl wearing white shirt and white hijab with sunglasses in various pose while seating on the wooden chair. Shutterstock. https://www.shutterstock.com/image-photo/beautiful-malay-girl-wearing-white-shirt-1503068691 and https://www.shutterstock.com/image-photo/beautiful-malay-girl-wearing-white-shirt-1503068711

SHVETS production. (2021, March 8). Female talking with psychologist during session. Pexels. https://www.pexels.com/photo/female-talking-with-psychologist-during-session-7176296/

Subbotina Anna. (n.d.). Winking sexy model Girl holding funny paper crown on stick isolated on white background. Shutterstock. https://www.shutterstock.com/image-photo/winking-sexy-model-girl-holding-funny-403636060

Svetography. (n.d.). Moon and sun girls. Shutterstock. https://www.shutterstock.com/image-photo/moon-sun-girls-380062678

tamarabegucheva. (n.d.). Attractive stylish woman in a red dress sitting on the table and holding his tie in front of a man in a suit, looking him in the eye. Shutterstock. https://www.shutterstock.com/image-photo/attractive-stylish-woman-red-dress-sitting-476409535

Tiểu Bảo Trương. (2019, July 7). Cute woman in a pink dress on pink background. Pexels. https://www.pexels.com/photo/cute-woman-in-a-pink-dress-on-pink-background-7569810/

Tiểu Bảo Trương. (n.d.). Ao dai asian model asian woman. Pixabay. https://pixabay.com/photos/ao-dai-asian-model-asian-woman-6182821/

Vlada Karpovich. (2021, May 27). Woman in red corporate attire standing behind the table while seriously looking at the camera. Pexels. https://www.pexels.com/photo/woman-in-red-corporate-attire-standing-behind-the-table-while-seriously-looking-at-the-camera-8367798/

Made in the USA
Las Vegas, NV
31 October 2023

79897588R00075